The Survival

LISA WB

Published in 2013 by FeedARead.com Publishing – Arts Council funded
Copyright © **Lisa Whenham-Bossy MBPsS HSC**

First Edition

A CIP catalogue record for this title is available from the British Library.

Acknowledgements

I would like to thank all of the people who have given me support for helping me to write *The Survival*. I am grateful for the professional service from Rebecca Keys for helping to edit the book. Thank you to Aileen Sneddon for help with the cover design.

A humble thank you to all those who have read and supported my books, and to those who have sent messages and who have also inspired me.

A huge thank you to all the medical staff involved with my recovery. A special thank you to Maggie Bodington, my diabetic nurse, and to Fahreen Dhanji, my GP. I would also like to thank the professionals who have read my books and who have taken the time to give me feedback.

I will be eternally grateful to Dr Trevor Friedman, who has restored my faith in people, and through his dedicated professionalism, patience and care has helped me to recover to a stage I never thought I would reach. I would also like to thank him for not only contributing to this book, but for accepting an ongoing friendship which I feel privileged to have.

A heart-warming thanks to family and friends, to Pauline Menzies-Gow for showing me what genuine friendship is, likewise to Sam Hessin and Gail Coleman who never fail to make me smile.

I could not have written this book without the support from Patrick, my husband who I love dearly, and from my two children Joëlle and Tanguy who I am so proud of and love so much.

I hope that this book helps to demonstrate just a little, that there can be a way back from the dark.

FOREWORD

I was very pleased to be asked to write a foreword for Lisa's new book. I was Lisa's psychiatrist and figure as 'Dr Lynn' in her previous book – A Fine Line. I treated Lisa for almost 20 years; an extremely long time to see any patient in the National Health Service. I remember during her therapy sessions, Lisa telling me that she intended to write a book about her life and treatment. We often discussed the purpose of the book and what she hoped to gain from writing it. She never expected it to have the success it has achieved and that so many thousands of people would read it and find it of interest and benefit to them.

The reason that the account of her journey over the years and the therapy she received is important and interesting is that Lisa gives a fascinating insight to her experience of undergoing treatment; both the positive and negative aspects. The book is not meant to be a scientific, rational account of someone who has been severely abused disclosing her experiences and this leading to a cathartic moment of insight and cure. Lisa describes that whilst intellectually understanding that she suffered abuse, she struggles with the conflict of accepting that she was abused by people she believed were caring or loving at the time. The book describes how difficult it can be to overcome the resistance to change. Lisa's account of her treatment illustrates that whilst insight is obviously important in getting better, the process of being cured and being content is much more complex and tortuous.

The book also provides great insight into the experience of being a psychiatric patient; particularly as an inpatient on a busy ward. She describes how care was or was not provided. As a Consultant Psychiatrist, I did not always know what really happened in the ward at night times and weekends when there were fewer senior staff around. Her account was of such significance that it became required reading for senior managers in our mental health organisation. Lisa was also asked by the Chief Executive to offer advice about the nursing care and organisation for a new all-female ward. This illustrates the importance of her account of her experiences.

The book is also a very personal account from Lisa. I may disagree with some of her understanding or interpretation of events. The value of the book comes from her honesty in writing what she experienced and believed at the time. The reader has the opportunity to hear Lisa's voice over the years; her struggles to unearth the truth about her life. It is not a simple story with an easy conclusion; it is all the more powerful and realistic for that. It will obviously be of interest to people who have suffered abuse in their own lives, but also to a wider audience of anyone interested in understanding how an intelligent young woman can be seduced by abusers and the huge struggle to undo the harm caused.

Dr Trevor Friedman BSc MB BS FRC Psych

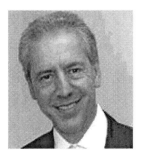

CHAPTER ONE – SOWING THE SEED

"Write a sequel!"

"Why?"

"You know why."

I laughed and looked over at my friend as we watched our children play basketball. She wasn't laughing, but looked deadly serious. I bit my lip, thinking how my book called *A Fine Line – A Balance to Survive* had suddenly become a number-one bestseller in several categories on Amazon in both the UK and USA stores, and Sam wasn't the first friend to suggest I write a sequel.

My first book was based on my life, which was colourful as it had been tainted with serious child abuse. Some people might question the word 'colourful', as many who experience child abuse have an inner sensation about the dark, or 'the black'. It was a dark area to enter, and to some 'shut doors'. Unfortunately to those that have experienced child abuse 'shutting doors' isn't always possible.

***

Flashback:

I woke up feeling hot, the trickling sweat seeping down the centre of my developing body. It caused a little pool in my navel. I moved to escape my bedraggled state and was pushed back. A hand smeared the sweat across my midriff and crept down between my legs, and then as my growing ribs bore the pressure of a huge weight, I was overcome by the black.

The freezing cold water caused me to gasp, and my knees gave way. Strong arms held me back up, and then the shower came to a halt. I was swaddled in a thick warm bath towel and carried back down the stairs to the large sofa in the living room. She placed me in the corner of the sofa and I huddled, feeling life flow back through my body as the warmth seeped through my soul. Next a big mug of steaming hot chocolate was placed in front of me on top of the thick wooden coffee table. I sat back; I hadn't got the strength to hold the mug. My head rested against the cushions, and I stared at the television without really seeing what was on.

Sometime later she walked me home; often I would have to sit down on the kerb just to get my breath back. Home was where I lived with my parents and two sisters, ten minutes around the corner from her house. On nights like this, the ten minutes could have been hours. She left me at the gate, and as the moon slithered out from behind the cloud I crept around the side of our bungalow and let myself in quietly through the back door.

***

My consultant liaison psychiatrist Dr Lynn had been seeing me since 1994, and we had built a decent professional relationship. I respected him greatly, yet this did not stop me from challenging some of his views. Sometimes his challenges did make me rethink, and in other cases I still thought he was way off the mark. Whatever the outcome, I believe he and his team had built a framework that helped support my needs, and gave me a vital lifeline that was permanently activated and helped keep me alive.

Many people who knew me would have been shocked at this statement. Why would I need a lifeline when I had a fantastic family consisting of my two children Jo Jo, who was now a very active fourteen-year-old, my son Tee Jay who was maturing into a sensible lad of twelve, and of course my Swiss husband Joseph, who had stuck with me through thick and thin, and even now we still had our sticky patches. I believed marriage wasn't handed to you on a plate and that you had to work at it. We seemed to have worked very hard recently, but we were still on the same plate.

Due to the events of my past, I been diagnosed as a major depressive and also suffered from post-traumatic stress disorder. Triggers could set off flashbacks, and due to the complex nature of the mind it was usually when I was at my most relaxed or enjoying life that I could be hit by a crisis. A crisis could range from feeling distressed to being suicidal; the intensity varied and was unpredictable. The nature of the illness didn't help either; many people who hadn't suffered trauma could not understand the depth of the illness. It was not a matter of pulling yourself together, as the thoughts came from the subconscious and were 'penetrating' or 'intrusive' as the professionals would call them. It was hard to explain, but by the time you wanted to block the thought it had already happened, and it was how you managed it after that counted. But by this time the damage could have already been planted. Also, as with other traumatic incidents, suppression may have helped at the time of the incident, but the consequence was that the suppressed feelings, images and thoughts could enter the consciousness at any time, causing instability and anxiety.

I judged myself fortunate that life could be pretty normal in between the crises, but even to hit the normal I had to be occupied at a high rate 24/7 except for the time when I slept, and even then nightmares and flashbacks were regular visitors. Thanks to Dr Lynn, the episodes between the crises were now longer and the intensity of each crisis lower. But the unpredictability still lay just around the corner, and only recently I had an episode where I was fighting to stay alive and not to act on suicidal thoughts.

Over time what I had learned was that when a crisis struck I would have approximately two weeks of fighting the intensity and then it would go. The experience of learning that the distress would go after two weeks, giving a week or two, would help enormously. The downfalls were that I would be physically and mentally exhausted afterwards, as to fight for the two weeks to stay alive and not to self-harm meant keeping myself so busy and occupied that it was impossible to stop. This meant multi-tasking at a rate that most women would find impossible. Men would not know the meaning of the word – or to be fair, my husband wouldn't. My children helped me enormously as I tried to think of them when fighting the bad thoughts. Even then at times I had to get away from the kids, not because I wanted to but because I didn't want them to know their mother was having a difficult time.

I first met Dr Lynn after a car 'accident', although it was still questionable whether it had been planned. I had lost my memory and been referred to see him. It had taken several years of me just sitting there in his consulting room before I would talk. During those consultations I would hand him a piece of paper with scraps of my writing on it. Even then some days I was hesitant to pass him the paper. I felt suspicious and I was very wary.

Dr Lynn was very tall, and he could easily have come across as imposing. He didn't, and he would sit back in his chair, cross his legs and wait very patiently. He would study or read the pieces of paper, if I passed any, and quietly comment or ask a question. In the earlier years I could never answer. I would just sit and make facial expressions.

Self-harm is a sensitive subject, and one again that some people have a problem getting their head around. I thought I understood it as a coping mechanism. I knew when I was distressed and suffering from intrusive thoughts the only way to block them was to self-harm. I had tried all the other ways – watching television and reading – but these would not come close to taking any edge off. The act of self-harm served as a diversion, and although temporary could give life-saving seconds. The other side of self-harm, in my opinion, was that it could become addictive, as in the act of carrying it out the endorphins and chemical changes in the brain could give an adrenalin rush so high that it gave out pleasure. This explanation I could understand, as anyone so distressed that they want to end their life to stop the pain may turn to self-harm where the diversion, although ugly, was life-saving. The part I didn't understand, and still don't, is that I self-harmed before I was even in my teens.

***

I was in the bathroom. Mum and Dad were in the kitchen, my sisters were around the house and I suddenly looked hard at myself in the mirror. I was told I was a pretty girl with dark hair, very dark eyes and a dark complexion. The adults would call me attractive, but at that age I wasn't sure what it meant. All of a sudden I wanted to hit myself so hard. I was a very tough tomboy who would prefer to kick a football around the garden with the boy from next- door than to play any other game. I was also very strong, and in a second or so I had given myself a black eye. I just raised my right hand and aimed purposely for the cheekbone. On the first impact my clenched knuckles caught it and a bump appeared straightaway. I wasn't satisfied and repeatedly thumped my face until I suddenly realised that I could only see my cheek out of that eye. I could see with my good eye that it was puffy and swollen. I quickly left the bathroom and made my way into my bedroom. My heart was racing and I was trying already to think of an excuse to my bruise. I worked it out and walked into the kitchen.

Mum was making some sandwiches and was leaning over the bread board. Dad turned round from the kitchen sink, tea towel in hand, and suddenly whistled. "What have you done to your face?"
Mum turned round, breadknife in her hand. She placed it down and walked over to me.

"I caught the edge of the table as I went to pick my book up."
I went to walk out of the room. "Come here, darling," Mum called me over.

She picked up the butter and then with her finger rubbed some butter onto my bruise. "The grease will help the swelling," she said.
I walked back into the bathroom and looked into the mirror, I was so pleased with the effect of the butter: the blue had darkened and the grease emphasised the bruising. Satisfied, I went and picked up my book.

***

I reflected back and thought hard, but it made no difference: I hadn't a clue why I had wanted to do that when I was younger. It was a significant event, as I had written about it in my first book. My mum and dad were respectable people, and both worked hard to bring their family up in the

10

correct manner. I admit I found it extremely hard to accept the fact that I was adopted, especially when my younger sister was born a couple of years after me, and my mum was over the moon. She never meant to show favouritism, but it shone from all corners, and my younger sister thrived in that sunlight. She was very out-going, popular and fun. I loved my sisters, but both had extremely different principles and morals to me. I was so overjoyed when I had my own two children, as for the first time I could look at my family and try to see a resemblance from me both mentally and physically. But even when I had my own two children and was happily married, I still suffered from flashbacks.

***

```
  My most consistent flashback:
  I woke up sweating and through my window I could hear
the dustbins rattling. I could see a figure climbing over
them trying to get to the window. He had short hair, pale
jeans and trainers. He was running towards me. I tried to
get up to move but I couldn't. It was as if my brain had
detached from my body. I could now hear his heavy
breathing and I screamed a silent scream. I fought hard
and heard a crash. I sat up, wide awake, and my lampshade
was on the floor. The wind blew the curtains gently and
the stars shone brightly. I climbed out of bed and looked
through the window: there was a field and the cows were
in – no dustbins, no man. I sighed and jumped back into
bed. I lay awake for a while thinking.
```

This flashback was a regular occurrence. Each time the man came and each time I didn't see his face.

***

My book was written on auto-pilot, and I kept myself distanced. Even to this day I argue with my consultant that it was written about someone else. We – that is, Dr Lynn and I – have this argument. He states that the book is false as it gives the reader the impression that I have dealt with the past and moved on. I believe that different readers will perceive it in various ways. The feedback that I have received is that people think I have moved on but still have a way to go. I did not plan the book – I just had a burning desire to write my story and to get it onto paper. I read many books about child abuse before I wrote mine, and always compared the book I was reading to my life. Each book I read has been significant, as each is individual with different meanings and messages. The end result was that the book was self-published, which was a disadvantage for a paperback, as the retail price was high, and although it was available online through all major bookshops the actual book was not on the shelf. So I set up a website to try to sell it and I was fortunate to gain an endorsement from a leading professor of biological psychology. His endorsement gave me great motivation, as he recognised the book as significant for its insights into child abuse and its consequences and the ambiguous psychiatric care at the hospital. I had an idea and wrote to the local Chief Executive of the NHS Partnership Trust. My luck was in, as he turned out to be a very caring man who deeply believed in better conditions for the Trust. He also recognised the significance of the book and also gave it a positive endorsement. I then used these endorsements and managed to receive praise from the British Psychology Society for the book and gain amazing support from many different professionals involved in child abuse-related issues.

When the book was published, many people were quite shocked and of course it was the hot topic at the primary school where Tee Jay still went. It wasn't every day that your child's friend's mum was suddenly in the local papers for telling the world she was a survivor of long-term child abuse and of several murder attempts. It wasn't every day that the parent who had been standing next to you in the playground suddenly told the world she had been in a high-security psychiatric unit and had been sectioned. The leaves whistled and fluttered on the trees in the playground, and it wasn't due to the weather.

I weathered the storm: I walked up to the school as if nothing had happened and nodded and smiled as I had done for years. The friends who knew me stood possibly closer than usual, as if they were there to protect against the unknown. I wasn't sure how people would react, and if the vicious tongues would cut through the air. Surprisingly a few people came up and congratulated me on the book, and some later even gave positive reviews. I started to receive messages through the website, and to my surprise I had many professional experts such as solicitors who dealt with child abuse cases, social workers and nurses message me and thank me for the insight the book gave them.

It was 2011, and I had just got back from attending a parents' meeting at Jo Jo's school. I was very proud of my daughter, as teacher after teacher gave a glowing report. One of the teachers even interrupted to say a good word for Tee Jay, who was two years younger. I came home proud of both my two children. I decided to go to bed early and read my new Kindle that Joseph had bought me for Christmas.

I leaned back in bed, Kindle closed, and thought of my past. Was it really as ugly as people made it out to be? I had written my book and Dr Lynn had challenged me so much on this topic. I admit I felt guilty when people wrote 'a courageous lady', etc., and I even received a message on Facebook telling me I was an amazing lady. I laughed at this one and wrote back, 'Well, I try my best'. I was joking, of course, and it was bizarre, as part of me felt sad. Dr Lynn challenged my thoughts, saying it was crazy that I could write this book and receive messages from people and still deny it happened to me. I knew where he was coming from, but it was just like that: all that had happened in the past and even today I can't write that it all happened 'to me'. It still seemed like another world, and that it had happened to someone else. I could tell people I had written a book, and it was true. Yet I couldn't verbally link things together. I was honest with people. I wasn't psychotic or round the bend, but I think this was all to do with denial, which sounds trivial, but denial has great depth, and I believed from what Dr Lynn had taught me that because of the denial I still suffered from trauma, unpredictable flashbacks and intense suicidal periods.

Sitting in bed writing this, I felt another pang of guilt. My daughter Jo Jo had come upstairs as well, and she was lying in Joseph's place writing on her computer to her friends. Joseph was downstairs watching his favourite programme and Tee Jay, bless him, had gone to bed. Why, I asked myself, why couldn't I admit to myself that…?

I couldn't even go there again, and my mind had blocked. I wondered whether it would have an effect if I started describing her, one of the people in the past. Then I stopped myself: that was like playing with fire and so dangerous. Triggers could set off my illness.

Even writing this I was learning and reflecting. In my other book I described her so well, but it was on auto-pilot, although perhaps further on in this book I will be able to do so again. It wasn't just about her – I had been unfortunate enough to have been repeatedly, attacked, raped… by many different people. It was because I had been groomed at such an early age – twelve years old to be precise – and groomed to such an extent that I didn't even realise what was happening. My mind suppressed event after event.

CHAPTER TWO – SANDRA

Dr Lynn had done his best to explain to me about the effects of grooming and the devastating effect and consequences of it. I thought I understood, yet I was disappointed that some of the feedback from my first book was that people could not understand why Bridget didn't walk away, or tell someone, or how she just let it happen time and time again. In particular most men didn't understand at all, whereas quite a few females did understand. It was an effect of the grooming: Bridget had been groomed to such an extent and the events had happened so regularly that it was a way of life to her. She had her vulnerability increased and turned against her. Paedophiles are very clever, and they groom so that the child feels it is the paedophile who is the trusted one and that everyone else is the enemy. I could really relate this to Sandra, as she pointed out how my parents loved Denny more and managed to convince me that I had been treated unfairly. Reflecting back, I think she exaggerated and empathised so much that I was overwhelmed by the care she seemed to demonstrate for me. I was disappointed that in some of the reviews from my first book people – even those with mental health problems – clearly did not understand the effects of child abuse. Suppression and denial were not even considered, grooming was not understood, and despite the book being documented as a true story with considerable backing from some of the medics involved, some reviewers even thought Bridget was delusional in her descriptions of Sandra. Some of these reviews bruised and hurt me; I wouldn't be human if they didn't. I actually reflected on them and came to the conclusion that it proved a point about how uneducated people were relating to mental health. It highlighted the need for improved insight into and education about mental health issues. I did not blame the reviewers. To this day I believe that the appropriate people who could change the stigma about mental health, through promotion and education, need a push. They need a hard push, as they themselves would have to break through the Victorian stigma about mental health and they would also need persuading hard as it would cost money, and unfortunately mental health comes way down the ladder of priority. In writing this it is not surprising that child abuse is so widespread and misunderstood, as the powers that be do not do enough about it. It is also not just about the powers to be: people are scared to break rank and be out of the crowd. They are too scared to speak out even for their nearest and dearest, for they are embarrassed in their ignorance and would prefer to push mental health issues back into the Dark Ages.

***

As for Sandra, I recalled the days she helped me with my homework. I had rushed home from school, changed into my jeans and sweatshirt and cycled to her house. She had looked at my homework and chatted about how I got on at school that day.

***

```
The 'BLACK':
I was in her bed naked, my head in her pillows. I
couldn't move because her chest was in my face. She had
placed a nipple into my mouth, and I was being forced to
suck. She was pushing her breast in. Struggling to
breathe, I gasped. Her weight was overbearing. She was a
big lady, and I was petite for my age. She rubbed herself
up and down on me; the whole bed shook. It hurt, the
friction of her pubic hairs on my private parts burnt,
and then the sweat started to trickle down. Squelching
sounds were made as she pushed and panted. She penetrated
me with her fingers, nails razor-sharp. The black rescued
me and I woke up with the freezing water…
```

***

It is strange writing this, as I don't feel anything. I somehow knew it hurt, and yet I write this with numbness. I think some people will stop reading in disgust when the truth is described, yet how is child abuse to be prevented if people haven't the courage to read about the truth? Child abuse is disgusting and sickening, but it happens, and the words are not going to be pretty. Many readers of my previous book sent messages of thanks that at last they didn't feel alone. They felt better because they realised they were not alone, that others could also relate to their feelings. Mothers sent 'thanks' as they understood what their child had gone through. My first book received thousands of positive messages, with a few cruel reviews through mainly ignorance. It got knocked about for its grammar, and regrettably it deserved this criticism, as I was let down by a professional edit. Yet it was sad that many critics were blind to the significance of the message it portrayed. I was shocked at how tunnel-visioned some people are, because the book had helped so many, and to me if the book could help one person then it was valuable. I likened it to someone making an important speech with a stutter. Just because the person stuttered through the speech did not take away the

15

importance of the content. Yet I am glad that the appropriate medics and societies have recognised the significance of the book.

***

She praised me and helped me finish my homework. I felt high and really special as she had told me my homework was good. Sandra talked about my nan, who I loved dearly and was in her eighties. At one stage Sandra had moved in with her before she got her own house. Sandra spoilt my nan too: she took her out, helped decorate her house and improved the heating. I could only see Sandra in the eyes of someone being very caring and helpful.

My mum liked Sandra too, and it was my mum who first introduced her to the family. She brought her round one lunchtime, introducing her as her boss. Sandra was very clever and I think my dad initially liked her too.

It was Mum who first suggested that Sandra took me out for the day; I think she thought I stayed in too much. I enjoyed being at home and I loved the outdoor life. We had a massive garden approximately half an acre that ran alongside a babbling brook separated by a row of ten gigantic weeping willows. Mum and Dad bred cocker spaniels, so I was lucky to be surrounded by these lovely little dogs, and able to choose Judy, my golden cocker spaniel, as a thirteenth birthday present.

We lived in a bungalow that was nice, quite modest and enhanced by the garden that was so well looked after that we could have charged people to look around. We had a vegetable garden, screened by a ten-metre-long privet hedge that was about eight feet high which Dad always had a job to trim back. The vegetable garden was well organised, with neat rows of cabbages, garden peas, beans, and potatoes. Dad also grew prize chrysanthemums with flower heads the size of a plate. A large area of the garden was lawn that was maintained as well as a bowling green. Dad was a dedicated gardener, and the lawnmower left regimented rows. My favourite spot was the old apple tree at the bottom. It was a great shape for climbing, and both I and my younger sister Denny enjoyed clambering to the top.
Denny was born in 1963 and she too was quite a tomboy. She had long blonde hair, freckles, bright blue eyes and our mum's smile. She was fit in every possible way; she could run faster than me, climb and jump higher and was a clothes size smaller. However, I was the stronger of the

two of us, and could compensate where it mattered. Jane was born in 1958 and she was the opposite of Denny and me. While we wore jeans and trainers, Jane would wear her best clothes whatever the occasion and spent time lounging around, reading, smoking and doing anything with the least exertion possible. Mum used to call her the Queen, and at times it caused problems. Mum would shout out sometimes, "This isn't a hotel!". She would get fed up with the lack of help. I got so fed up with my sister's laziness and my mum being at her beck and call that I started to help. I didn't like being a witness to my sister using my mum, and I started to visit Sandra more often.

Sandra would not only spoil me but she would teach me a lot of new practical skills. Her dad was a professional plumber and also highly skilled in the building trade. He was nice to me and I loved going round to Sandra's house to put my new lessons into place. I helped plaster the walls, build a partition wall placing the plasterboards, rewired (which was of course professionally checked), and build a stone fireplace. I learned to paint; brick lay, and hang wallpaper and so much more. It became regular routine to visit whenever I could, and especially stay around there at weekends.

Sandra's dad would be there most weekends and I liked him a lot. Sandra's parents bought one of Judy's puppies; she was a black cocker spaniel and very beautiful. I visited Sandra's parents' house often. The nice thing was that they also welcomed my nan with big open arms.

My family got fed up with me singing the praises of Sandra and her parents, and I had to be careful what I said. My mum also got very upset at me going out every possible moment to see Sandra. By the time I reached my teens, I was convinced that Sandra was the best person I had ever met. I was still best friends with Susanne, who I had met at infant school and been friends with since the age of five. The problem with Susanne's friendship was that she had a demanding mum, who was lovely but quite needy, and Susanne did not have a lot of spare time. She also let me down often when I was expecting to meet up, as kids do, and I would end up waiting hours and she wouldn't turn up. I therefore turned to Sandra more.

Sandra became a mixture of an older sister and a mum, although there were only twelve years' difference between us. As I grew to know her better, it was as if our roles changed. She would become very depressed and talk non-stop about her fiancé, who tragically dropped dead playing football. She would pull the heavy red velvet curtains closed, dim the lights and play Simon & Garfunkel's *Bridge Over Troubled Water* repeatedly. She would talk about the twins that she and her fiancé wanted to have, and she would also play *Tommy* by The Who. She would turn to cuddle me and tell me that the twins were going to have dark hair like mine and have dark eyes and would look like me. She would be crying and I would feel uncomfortable, unsure how to help. I would feel distressed, but I felt I had to be strong, as I had rarely seen a grown-up cry.

***

Flashback:
Wet tears rolled down, dripping onto my shoulder. My heart was pounding, and the pill bottle lay tipped up. Paracetamol was scattered everywhere. She clung to me like a young baby, face desperate. I felt helpless. 'Ring your mum. Tell your mum,' I half whispered. Scared, I felt responsible and alone. She shook her head violently, clinging to me more, grip tightening. The brown cover pulled over me and hands tore at my clothes. I froze. I suddenly couldn't move. The tears ceased, the panting became louder and louder, and suddenly she thrust so hard…

This time I came to in a pool of water. It was freezing cold, and as I tried to focus I realised I was in a heap on the shower floor. She wasn't there; I crawled off the base and just lay out of reach of the cold water. I closed my eyes and the black came again…

***

One day I was at Susanne's house, which was not far from the school. It was a small bungalow situated on the corner of a housing estate, with bright yellow curtains. Chatting to Susanne's mum, I looked out of the window and caught sight of Sandra's car parked a few hundred yards away. I briefly wondered what she was doing, then forgot about it. Susanne got on well with Sandra, but was a bit apprehensive when Sandra lost her temper. I was used to the tantrums, the slamming of doors and tears, non-stop smoking and ranting. Susanne looked nervous and went quite white the first time Sandra lost it in her presence.

***

This time I was at school and we were in the playground. We were playing a ball game with the lads, and I had gone to retrieve the ball, which had rolled onto a drain near the school gates. As I bent to pick up

18

the ball, I looked out of the gates and down the road. I was surprised to see Sandra's white Volvo parked, with her sitting behind her wheel. She had obviously been watching the game. Funny, I thought, then I realised it was her lunch break at work and presumed she had just arrived on the off-chance in case she would get to see me. I threw the ball hard into the crowd and forgot about Sandra as the school bell rang, an indication that dinner time was over.

* * *

Although I spent most of my time with Sandra in her house, she also spoiled me and took me shopping and out to places I hadn't been to before. I remember going to a place called Woburn Abbey and falling in love with the animals. We were driving through an area where the bears walked around freely when steam started coming out from the bonnet of the car, and Mum, who was with us, started to laugh. We weren't laughing five minutes later when the car broke down and a monkey sat staring through the windscreen at us whilst chewing at the windscreen wiper. Luckily we followed the rules and sat there and honked the horn, and soon the rangers managed to get the car going again. This time we drove without stopping. At other times Sandra also took my nan out; we had fun and it was great to see my nan laugh.

* * *

Flashback:

"Where are we going?" My hands clung to my seatbelt tightly, and I looked across at Sandra. I was worried, as it was getting late and I should have been home for 10.30pm, but instead of driving home, Sandra was driving at a fast rate across Leicester. She eventually pulled up alongside the road. The rain pelted down, and I shivered as I clambered out of the car behind her. She hadn't bothered to put her cigarette out, and it hung limply out of her mouth. She walked on in the rain and I followed.

I didn't know where we were, but it was a quiet spot and no traffic had gone by. I could hear the drone of the motorway and as we walked on I suddenly realised we were approaching a bridge that crossed the motorway. Sandra walked up to the edge and leaned over with her elbows resting on the railings. I tapped her on her shoulder. It made no difference: she stared out over the motorway, fag ash dropping onto the rushing traffic below. I dug my hands into my jeans pockets as if searching for comfort. I walked to and fro. It was freezing cold, sort of misty, and she just stood there. I walked over and tapped her again; this time she angrily shrugged her shoulders to ward me off. I looked around helplessly, but there was not a soul in sight. "Sandra," my voice seemed a whisper against the roar below. "Sandra." It still came out softly, yet inside I was screaming in desperation. Her response was to lean heavily over and gaze at the busy motorway. The wind whipped round my shoulders and its bitter bite nipped at my nose. "Sandra!" This time I was so loud that her eyes flinched, and for a moment I thought she was going to acknowledge me. She didn't, and I turned away feeling dismal. My fingers clawed at my thighs through my pockets, my toes burned through the cold, and I nearly hobbled in my torn-up trainers to reach up to her. "Please," I pleaded as I tugged at her sleeve. "Come on. We need to get away from here." She looked through me as if I wasn't there. My mind was racing. She often talked about ending it, and I had seen the tantrums and felt the despair. Now I couldn't feel anything; I was numb, shocked, and felt the weight of the world on my shoulders.

I hovered like a falcon seeking its prey. I was ready to swoop and pounce, I was so hoping someone would come by. I wanted the warmth of the car, but most of all I wanted to be in my own bed at home. Safe.

It was after midnight when I eventually arrived home. Sandra had at last turned and driven home like a robot. I crept in, scared that Mum or Dad might wake up and I would be in big trouble for being late. My luck was in: I could hear Dad snoring from their bedroom as I tiptoed through to my bedroom.

***

I can look back now and realise how needy Sandra appeared to be, this made me feel more powerless and trapped as I often felt so sorry for her wanting to end her life.

CHAPTER THREE – HOME LIFE

I woke up early. Joseph was still sleeping, and I could hear Jo Jo up, which was unusual. Tee Jay was still in bed, and that was normal as it took ages to get him up. I made myself a cup of tea and went to look at the computer for any emails. Jo Jo was just coming out of the shower.

"Morning," she said as she towel-dried her hair.

"Morning, darling." We embraced and she went back upstairs as I disappeared into our kitchen. I let Amba and Asti, our two dogs, out and fussed over the four cats as they trailed in one by one from the corridor. I could hear Bella, our newest addition, meowing from the shower room. At fourteen weeks old she wasn't allowed out into the garden. I emptied the dishwasher and made my tea and strolled into my little study.

My computer came on and I read my emails and then disappeared back to the kitchen to make Joseph a coffee. He usually brought me a cup of tea in bed every morning. He came downstairs to drink his coffee and he switched the news on the television. Most early mornings were taken up by making sure the kids got up on time for school. Jo Jo usually spent ages on her appearance, and Tee Jay would spend all morning in the paddock with the hens and ducks if we allowed him. However well we tried to be prepared, both Jo Jo and Tee Jay would suddenly lose something or remember they were supposed to get something signed. I would drive both kids and the neighbours' child to school every morning, and on Tuesdays I dropped them off where they had to walk a little further to school, as I had to see my GP at 8.30am.

I was very fortunate to have a lovely, understanding GP called Dr Dhanji, who I got on so well with that it was like going to visit one of my friends. We could both have a laugh even when we were having to check over the more serious side of my medical problems. She was extremely professional and efficient, and I suppose because of this I knew I could relax a little as she was so good. It was not often your doctor would give up her dinner hour to accompany you to see a diabetic nurse who you were just so anxious about seeing that you did not want to step over the threshold into her office. I first refused to see my diabetic nurse when I was diagnosed as diabetic earlier last year. It was Dr Dhanji who persuaded me, and on the initial meeting I swear the diabetic nurse was more anxious than me. I was lucky because she turned out to be a charming lady called Maggie, who was also very professional and caring, and after a few visits I started to relax as I grew to understand her and the illness. Another bonus was that I could also have a good laugh with Maggie, so our sessions were still enjoyable even when I was still trying to learn how to look after myself. I initially started on medication, but after a while it had no effect and I learned to take insulin. I disliked the injections but liked the flexibility of being able to adjust the insulin to my changing needs. Maggie was very patient and taught me a lot.

It was actually also a relief to gain some energy back. I had accepted that my extreme tiredness was due to my age, when the insulin started to work and my sugar levels started to normalise my energy returned.

When my book *A Fine Line – A Balance to Survive* was published I was initially concerned about the potential effect it could have on Jo Jo and Tee Jay. I did not take the decision to publish my book lightly, and I asked for advice from the medical professionals who looked after me. I also believed that Tee Jay and Jo Jo could absorb certain issues easier as children than when they were adults. I decided to tell them both that I had a book published about my life and that although when I was younger I had some nasty events happen to me, it was in the past and I was OK now. I also highlighted that the book may help other people. When I was lying on the sofa with Jo Jo, I turned round to look at her. "Can I tell you about my book, as I would rather you know about it from me than other people?" Jo Jo turned to look at me.

"You know my book is about me and my past?" I said.

She nodded. "Well, when I was younger I had some people try to hurt me and do some nasty things. I also survived some murder attempts." I hesitated and looked at her. She was expressionless. I continued as gently as I could. "You know I was in the psychiatric hospital for some time and Dr Lynn looked after me?" I waited and she nodded. "Well, it sounds silly, but some people may try to make fun of that because I was in a psychiatric unit, but if they did start to make fun, it is because deep down they haven't a clue what it is all about." Jo Jo had sat up now and was looking intently at me. "What I am trying to say is that if people make fun and laugh, who knows more about that situation, you or them?"

"Me," said Jo Jo.

"And do you think it was funny?"

"No." She shook her head.

"Well, just remember who knows best." I smiled at her, and she cuddled up to me.

"I will have nightmares now," she said. I sighed, as that was the last thing I wanted to hear.

"Why?" I asked.

"Because people tried to kill you." She squeezed my hand hard.

"OK, let's look at it this way," I said. "Am I any different now than I was five minutes ago before I told you anything?" Jo Jo shook her head. "Well, why make anything different? That was a long time ago and I am exactly the same as I was five minutes before I told you. Think about it." Jo Jo smiled and so did I. *Phew*, I thought to myself. *One hurdle down, another to go.* I didn't explain as much to Tee Jay as he was that much younger, and I didn't think the situation would arise. He just understood that Mummy had written a book about her past and that some people had thanked her and that the book was helping people. I realised I could tell my children it was about me as I knew they wouldn't read it and it didn't feel real, yet having to confront the situation with Dr Lynn or any other adult was a challenge too far.

The book was helping people, but it had its drawbacks, and to me it was from the people I least expected it from.

My past had largely been supressed, as is the nature of child abuse, so when I was eventually admitted into hospital for therapy, it came as a massive shock to my mum. I lost my lovely dad in 1999 to pancreatic cancer, and he died never knowing the truth about my past. I was still in denial when I went into hospital in 2001, and one of the consequences was that a lot of the past was still hidden or not revealed. Once the book was out, I realised that I had wanted my family to read it and then mend the hurt by giving me a big hug, telling me they never realised about the past, and that everything would be OK. That didn't happen, and the dream ending in my book of being united with my mum and two sisters didn't happen either.

My mum had a job to even acknowledge the book. Denny, my younger sister, did not want to read it, but later was happy for me that the book was doing so well. My older sister Jane took it as the opportunity she was always looking for and broke off contact with me completely Her reaction after reading the book was to reunite with him and go on holiday with him, and to not only break contact with me but to also cut off contact with my children. As the book had revealed my brother-in-law's attempts to kill me, I was just a bit taken back that she wouldn't acknowledge anything was his fault. Our estrangement obviously upset my mum, and she asked me to give Jane time. To my surprise I replied, "Mum, sorry, but for the first time in my life it's a relief not to have the pressure of trying to make up under false pretences. I don't want to make up; it's a relief that she is out of my life. I will always love her, but her principles and morals are so different to mine. We have never got on." Mum sighed and looked at me, looking exasperated, but for once I felt I had done the right thing. Joseph backed me and I knew from how Jane had recently taken up living in my mum's house and taken advantage of mum that I had done the right thing. It was very difficult for Mum and I to be firm enough to throw her and her children out from Mum's home, but knowing it was the only way she would find herself somewhere new to live after her husband had left her homeless, we continued to be cruel to be kind. She did find somewhere to live. I didn't cut off her children, and I still bought them birthday and Christmas presents despite my sister cutting Jo Jo and Tee Jay off. I also welcomed them into my house. I think it was a relief for Jane, as she had never liked me from when we were little and had spent years trying to criticise me or bring me down in front of anyone. When she found out that the bank manager had raped me, her response had been, 'It's about time it happened to her'. Jane and her husband also set me up with a blind date. When I met him over dinner at their house, I took an instant dislike to the guy. It was a few weeks later when they told me that he had just come out of prison for rape and he had also been in for grievous bodily harm. Jane also used to ring me up daily when I was expecting Jo Jo and always asked, 'What will you do if there is something wrong with the baby?'

***

My family's reaction to the book hurt me. I had wanted my mum to read it and feel some sort of empathy, and I felt hurt that my younger sister Denny was more interested in being angry at me letting one of her friends read it than acknowledging the content inside. Obviously Jane just denied it all, and used it as an excuse to cut me out of her life. Dr Lynn talked it through with me, saying, "Why, why would you expect anything different?" He actually thought it was a good learning curve for me. I didn't blame Jane;, it put her in a very difficult position as she still loved her husband and of course he was the dad of her two children. I didn't blame Mum either, and considering the content, her age and the shock of it all, I think she handled it quite well. Both she and Denny have accepted the book, yet still hate it and don't want people to read it. I don't expect more than that from them. Inside I feel a little bitter, but no one is perfect and how can people judge unless they are in the same situation? I am still amazed at the response from people and the kindness they have shown. The fact that the book has also been seen as being useful helps to change the negatives of the past into positives. I also realised that if even I was still in denial over some of my past, it was wrong of me to expect my family to accept it. I also thought that just because they didn't acknowledge my past didn't mean that they didn't care; it just meant they were incapable at that time of managing it in the way I wished them to.

CHAPTER FOUR – TRUST

Dr Lynn still challenged me a lot, and it was only the other week that we were talking about trust. Although I had been seeing him for nearly seventeen years, I was still wary. I preferred to sit in the chair with the nearest access to the door, so that if he made a sudden move I could jump. Last week we were in a different room to usual, but I had been in it before and I still didn't like it. This time when I entered the room, the desk had been swung round to be adjacent to the wall instead of coming out from it. The result was that there was plenty of space on the wooden floor. It gave me a flashback – not a heavy one, but everywhere I looked I was in the past.

***

Flashback:
The bank manager had taken me up to the small room above the bank where all the files were kept. Access was through a loft door, and as soon as he followed me through, he whipped the door shut fast, grabbing my ankle and causing me to fall on top of the door. He laughed. "We won't have to lock it, will we?" Before I had time to answer he was already pulling my skirt up over my head, hand reaching down under my underwear. I couldn't move. I was aware that he had pushed himself inside me and he was now pushing up and hard and was panting heavily. I tried to focus on the wooden floor, and then he had changed: it wasn't him, it was the vet, and this time he was pushing me over onto my front and I remember trying so hard to turn back but he wouldn't let me. I stared hard, aware Dr Lynn was asking me something, but it was weird, so weird. I could hear him but I could see the wooden floor, and I could feel the vet, now having turned me on my front, start to kneel and climb up the back of my legs. It was getting so desperate and just as he was about to enter me, my mind flashed back to her sharp nails…

***

I was swapping and changing images, and everywhere I looked I could see images that I did not want to see. In desperation I turned to Dr Lynn. "Soldiers when they come home from the war… do they… would they see…" I couldn't finish, as when I got worked up my sentences were stilted. I finally continued. "Would they see the battlefield? Would they see…"

My voice trailed off. Dr Lynn just sat there not saying anything, and then I felt stupid. "Sorry," I muttered. I looked around, but even before I started to look, I could still see the past shifting from one event to the next. I felt a bit shaken and I still did not like the big empty space on the floor. Dr Lynn challenged me on my thoughts about having to sit on the chair nearest the door. "Why, Bridget? What do you think I am going to do?"

"Well, it's not the same, is it, as you aren't going to do anything here as there are too many people about, and it's not the same as…" It was strange, as I was thinking that it wasn't like being alone in a house or building with someone, and if he wanted to do anything it would be difficult. Part of me rationalised, and deep down I knew it was OK because it was Dr Lynn, yet part of me was still terrified. In my eyes, people who were nice turned round and did that sort of thing. It happened to me every day for over twenty years, so could I be sure it wouldn't happen? The people who had abused me before turned out to be professional people: a vet, a bank manager, a policeman, my mum's boss, my brother-in-law… the list could have continued. I just felt safer when I was nearer the door. Dr Lynn spoke, "We will have to see another time if *I* can sit near the door." I wasn't sure if he was joking or being serious. He told me he would see me in a fortnight and I thanked him and left the building.

As I walked outside, the glare of the daylight hit me. It was a reminder of how dark and dismal it was inside. I could still smell the staleness of the air, and I was thankful for the small breeze that sent a paper bag flying into the sky. I looked up at the dark building and remembered a horrific event that had occurred whilst I was an in-patient at the hospital. I was so glad that Jo Jo and Tee Jay hadn't visited me that day.

***

I was laughing with Zena, a nurse who was accompanying me. As I was on level one, a nurse was supposed to be within a shoulder's length of me at all times. The nurses changed every hour. Zena and I had decided to go and sit in the enclosed courtyard area outside when the silence was broken by the sound of crashing glass just above my head, a whoosh that made me duck, and behind me a huge thud. Zena pushed me hard back through the doors onto the ward. Screams echoed around the building, and chaos flooded through. The tags had been pulled, and nurses ran through with doctors to the courtyard and the area was screened off. It was an agonising wait, and the thud seemed to echo time and time again. I had just felt the sensation of a weight fall from a level or another level up just behind me, and hadn't had chance to register what it was as I was pushed back inside. I then realised it was a person, and everyone was hovering and anxious. The doctors and nurses worked hard to save a life, but unfortunately it was not to be, and the ward was sombre.

***

It was incidents like this in the hospital that I had to cut out of my first book, but I felt they were still significant enough to be remembered. I still had flashbacks of that body crashing to the ground. This event, combined with a separate incident of a girl who had been moved next to my room trying to smash the room up, had a negative effect on me. It gave me illusions of a way out of the cage that I was trapped in. At the time it was worse than a mouse cage with a wheel, as to me this cage had no boredom relief and it also had inmates who could be damaging with their negative influences and lethal advice. One girl gave me advice about the proper way to slit your wrist, and to my horror the nurses confirmed she was right. There were also very aggressive inmates who could be dangerous, so I could not relax and was always on my guard. I still had flashbacks of the incidents where I smashed window after window and attempted to go through. The feeling of being institutionalised had a massive impact, and rationality was diffused.

***

It was February 2011, and I felt amazed and very humbled that my book was still number one in child abuse and several other categories on Amazon UK. I emailed one of the teachers at my children's school. I had met her several times, as she was the person in charge of Special Educational Needs. She had been very supportive to me when I first approached the school when Jo Jo was due to go there. She had also bought a signed copy of my book, so I did not have to explain as she was familiar with my problems and issues and how they sometimes had an impact on the children. I copied and pasted my book's rankings to her and wrote that I found it surreal. She answered back about rewards for being so brave. It was a comfort to me to know that I still had the support from various people who I had met through different aspects of my life.

***

I challenged myself on this book and asked Sam, my friend from basketball and the mother of my son's friend Tom, her opinion. Anyway, Sam replied, "I want to read your sequel, and so will many other people. Everyone will want to know what happened next and how you are doing. I can't wait to read it."

"Yes, but don't you think that's because you know me?" I argued back.

"No," Sam shook her head emphatically. "No, people will want to know. It's that sort of book, and your writing is so compelling that you just want to keep reading." I laughed at her and pondered. I still wasn't sure, but deep inside I knew I had so much more to tell. Sam's son Tom was a whizzkid at sport, and a keen boxer. The local paper had just written a piece about Tom

27

being the next Ricky Hatton, and I knew Sam felt very proud of him. I admired Sam, as she was bringing her four kids up on her own. We both sat back and continued to watch the basketball. It was a local club, and all the kids were so lucky to have a dedicated coach, Neil, and a club with a fantastic atmosphere. Andy also helped, and both men were good at coaching and giving the kids confidence and motivation. Both Tee Jay and Jo Jo loved to play basketball, and they had been selected to play in the club's teams. Tom played in the same team as Tee Jay, so it was nice as I could travel to Nottingham and see Sam there and share watching our children compete.

"Come on," Sam said as we were waiting for the kids to play their league game. "Tell me some more about the book."

"Which bit?" I asked, not having a clue.

"Any," Sam answered back. I hesitated, as the match had started and I wanted to watch Tee Jay play. Sam sat back, as she too wanted to watch the match. We both suddenly clapped like mad as Tee Jay scored. It was only seconds later when Tee Jay scored a three-pointer from outside the scoring zone. It was nice, as Tom was usually one of the top players and Tee Jay was playing like I had never seen him play before. The quarter ended and I took the chance to tell Sam about a time when I was in hospital that I had so wanted to write about in *A Fine Line* but had no room left for it.

***

"When I agreed to go into hospital, in a psychiatric ward, it was on a volunteer status and a predicted two-week stay. Neither I nor Dr Lynn realised the depth of the problems that would unfold. I had helped Joseph prepare his business accounts for the VAT, had sorted out enough food for the household and the animals, and literally planned for two weeks away. I knew the hardest task would be the separation from Tee Jay and Jo Jo, as every second would seem like hours. It turned out that every second seemed like days, and the two weeks turned out to be eight months. It also tore at me to say goodbye to my two dogs Amba and Jaz, as well as my four cats. Jaz was a rescued German Shepherd dog and she had a very unpredictable temperament so I asked Joseph to place her in some boarding kennels for her own protection as well as the children's. I knew deep down that she was becoming a problem as she kept escaping from our garden, and the more we tried to resolve the problem the more she tried to escape. It was a significant problem, as although she was well behaved, if trapped she could turn and become dangerous. I also talked about her with Joseph and we decided that if the kennels could find someone who would give her a good home we would let her go, on the grounds that the person was experienced and was clear what they were taking on This was not an easy decision, but I also wanted Jaz to have a happy life, as she deserved to be happy after her miserable start to life."

Lethal let-down.

I paused for breath. Sam had forgotten about the match and was listening to me intently. I continued.

"My mum volunteered to put it into writing and contact the kennels, and I felt at ease knowing Jaz would be safe and I could relax as I thought the problem was resolved. The last thing I expected was for Joseph to visit me whilst I was in hospital and give me the news he did.

Joseph hovered anxiously with a piece of paper in his hand, went to give it me, then took it away again. He muttered.

"I didn't know. I don't understand." He looked miserable, staring down at the floor. I watched him in alarm, with an awful feeling in my stomach. I felt sick and I hadn't even looked at the paper. I grabbed the paper off him and nearly fainted. It was an invoice from our vet for euthanasia: my dog had been put down without any notification or permission from me or Joseph. I kept conjuring images of them holding and trapping Jaz, and I knew she would have been terrified. I couldn't look at Joseph. I knew he felt upset by it as well. "Why?" I muttered. He shrugged his shoulders helplessly.

I felt so sick, yet also angry, upset and desperate. "If I wanted Jaz put down I wouldn't have paid for her to go to kennels, I would have asked the vet. What is going on? I want a solicitor."

Joseph grabbed my hand and squeezed tightly. "I don't know. I rang the kennels in Waltham, and the owner has been busy as her son was in a car accident. She hasn't come back to me."

It was some time later when I was on my own in hospital that I sank really low. I blamed myself, and thought I had let Jaz down. I picked up a piece of glass that I had hidden in one of the drawers, despite being accompanied by a level-one nurse who was more interested in her newspaper than me at the time. I lay on top of the bed with this glass pressing into my stomach. I was distraught and just wanted to cut. The situation was made worse by Lee, one of the nurses, who half laughed when he heard the news and seemed to be gloating."

Sam interrupted. "The bastard." I took a deep breath and carried on.

"I felt upset and sick, picturing my poor dog being put to sleep. Eventually Kim, one of the other patients, came to visit me. She was a registered GP, yet she was in hospital as she suffered from manic depression and at the moment she was quite high. She whispered an idea to me, and with the mood I was in it seemed a great idea. We had worked out that the end door of the courtyard wasn't always locked. This meant that if you walked into the courtyard from the ward, you could bypass the main ward doors that led out, and gain exit by this small door hidden in the corner, which was supposed to be locked. Neither Kim nor I was supposed to be allowed out. Kim wanted to go to Blackpool and she begged me to take her.

"I haven't a car," I protested to her as she tried to persuade me.

"We can take mine. We can get a taxi to my house and we can take my car. Please, Bridget, we will have so much fun." She fluttered her eyelashes and pulled a baby face.

I looked across at the nurse, who was sitting at my doorway as I was still on level one.

"Well, I am insured to drive other people's cars, but are you sure we will get out?"

"Look, I'll distract your nurse, then as soon as we're in the courtyard, don't look at me, just walk quickly up to the far door and walk out. Don't stop until you are out of the gates and meet me on the main road to the right." Kim nodded assertively. "We will go tomorrow morning, so be prepared." I watched her as she left the room. She was a tall girl with curly hair and glasses, and had certainly brightened up my days on the ward. Her high moods had caused her to act outrageously at times, flirting with Dr Lynn and the nurses and creating chaos. It was funny to witness, as she meant no harm and it was like being with a big kid.

The morning came and I skipped breakfast, not being hungry, and I still had my piece of glass in my pocket. It gave me comfort to know it was there. I had become so used to cutting as a self-harm method that I needed to keep a tool of any sort that could inflict a tear on my skin at the slightest motion."

Sam pulled a face. "Ooh you don't do it now, do you?" I shrugged and continued.

"My weapons were self-made, and in hospital I learned to adapt and use anything that I could get my hands on. I think if I had easy access I might not have been so desperate. My tools included ripped credit cards and cutlery, which I had learned the knack of breaking them behind my back at the second attempt of bending them. I had used my spare time in hospital to learn and adapt my actions and behaviour to the specific surroundings and context. I examined the cutlery in detail. I learned which type of fork would snap quickest, as some had thicker handles. I learned which spoon and knife would also snap easier. I could bend them so easily that even the anticipation of feeling the hot metal before it snapped would send my adrenalin rushing. I searched the cutlery tray and sometimes took two sets if the opportunity was right. Even the task of wrapping a spare towel or clothing around a mug before I smashed it became an art. Another patient taught me how to hold the mug at the correct angle, so that the slightest contact would send the handle flying off. Now as I fingered the glass I waited nervously for Kim to appear. She walked in at exactly 10.00am. We had planned that the medication trolley would be finished, but most of the nurses would still be clearing up. "Hi, Bridge," she said. "Come and see what Andrea and I did yesterday in the courtyard." I looked up to my nurse expectantly. She nodded, and I got up to follow Kim down the corridor into the reception area and out to the courtyard. I observed every person on my way through, and noted which nurses were where. My unsuspecting nurse followed us through to the courtyard. I hung back a little and hoped that Kim's idea would work. It did: she had engaged my nurse in conversation and was talking, and I was following them both to near the trough of plants. Then as Kim and my nurse went to look at the plant Kim had made a fuss about, I quickly turned direction and headed for the far door. I did not run but walked as quickly as I could. My nurse still followed Kim, who was chatting away about the trough. Once at the door I went through it slowly and quietly, and as soon as I was on the other side I ran as fast as I could out through the main reception, out through the double doors into the car park. I then ran like mad through the hospital gates and out onto the pavements. I didn't stop and ran until I reached where Kim had told me. I knew I was OK there as the nurses didn't continue that far if they were chasing or searching. All I had to do was to wait and hope that Kim would make it.

I shivered. I hadn't got my coat, as the nurse would have been suspicious. I used my time to look at the surroundings: there was an estate opposite and the gates and walls had been decorated with brightly coloured graffiti. Some of the flats above had little balconies, and many had clothes hanging from a line. My thoughts were interrupted by the sound of laughter, and Kim appeared. "Oh my God, you are in so much fucking trouble!" She laughed and clapped her hands together. "Come on. Let's go." We walked around the corner to a waiting taxi. Kim had planned this in detail. As we sat in the back, she related what had happened after I had left, speaking quietly as the taxi driver had the little window open. "I was trying not to laugh. Rachel carried on following me, and I was trying to make out that this plant had appeared out of nowhere. I leaned forward and asked her if she could see the roots, and she even bent forward to look. It was at that moment that she suddenly realised that you were not behind her and she panicked and pulled her tag." Kim started to cough as she laughed. "Rachel pulled her tag but went running back on the ward to see if you were there. The other nurses automatically followed her and they headed for your room. It was so easy for me: I just walked out as quickly as I could and headed in the opposite direction to the main building. I heard them all run the other way to the exit. I walked to the coffee shop and then made my way here. Look, I bought two muffins." She pulled out two squashed cakes from her pocket and passed me one. I took it although I wasn't hungry and I wasn't even enjoying this. I kept thinking of Jaz. The taxi driver dropped us off at Kim's home, and she let herself in, coming out five minutes later with her car keys. "You drive," she said, throwing the keys across to me. I felt nervous, but let myself into the driver's seat and opened the door for her. It was a sports car and I could feel the power of the engine as soon as my foot touched the throttle. We called in at the local garage to top up the petrol, and then headed north to Blackpool. Kim was laughing so much, and I tried to concentrate as I was driving on the motorway. "Be careful; don't attract attention. We don't want the police after us, do we?" Kim laughed. I looked in my mirror and decided to take it steady. I wasn't enjoying it, and I felt low, desperate and upset. In contrast, Kim was on a high and singing loudly in the passenger seat.

Three hours later we had booked ourselves into the pokiest little bed and breakfast, where I could smell the damp as we walked through the door. It was terrible, although Kim seemed to be happy. She bought a big purple curly wig at the fairground, and I had to laugh as she was a very tall lady, and so loud and bubbly that people turned round to look at us. We walked along the pier and Kim went straight for the fruit machines and started to play. My mobile phone rang and it was Joseph.

"Where the hell are you?"

I had never heard him so angry, and I hesitated, not knowing how to tell him. I bit my lip, looking at Kim scooping up her winnings, I moved away from an old man puffing black clouds of smoke next to me. I stood near the opening and looked out across the buildings to the sea. "I am in Blackpool," I whispered. "Kim arranged it."

"How is that going to help?" he said. "What about me and the children? When are you coming home?" The phone went dead. He hadn't been asking; he was shouting. I felt so miserable, I didn't know what to do, and I didn't want to go to the bed and breakfast place. It was a dirty hovel. Kim came over, asking, "What's up, doll?" She dug her hands in her pockets and brought out handfuls of coins, "Come on, have a go. Hurry up as I need a wee and a fag." I took a deep breath and thought, looking at the sea and listening to the screaming seagulls. I turned round to Kim.

"Sorry, I can't stay. It was a mistake and I need to get back." I could picture Jaz being held whilst she was injected and felt sick. I continued to explain.

"I feel responsible and want to let the ward know we are safe."

"Fine, don't worry about it. Take my car," replied Kim, smiling. I thought she was going to have a right go at me.

"I can't take your car. What about you?" I looked at her, and she was so high I knew I couldn't leave her. She started laughing, "I am fine. Ring the ward, and don't worry." While she wandered off to the nearest fruit machine, I rang the ward. Alec answered; I liked him. I couldn't speak and hesitated. He guessed, as I often couldn't speak when I was worked up. "Bridget, where are you?" He sounded concerned rather than angry. I hesitated and he again spoke. "Bridget, we are not angry with you. We know you are upset and we are just worried."

"I am in Blackpool with Kim."

"Kim? Is she alright?"

"She is very high, and she won't come back. I can't leave her. She wants me to drive her car, and I can't come back without her." I looked over my shoulder at Kim, who was singing and waving her hands in the air as she played the fruit machines. It was hard to imagine her as a GP, but I realised that she was ill at the moment and not her usual self. "Look, Bridget, get back here. Ask Kim to come too, but if she won't come you will have to leave her." Alec sounded determined.

"OK. I just wanted you to know that we were OK," I mumbled. I felt ashamed, yet I felt betrayed by all human beings, my dog was dead and it seemed no one could be trusted.

Kim was positive she wanted me to go and she refused to come back with me. "I am fine. Let me have some fun, please, Bridge. I don't want to go back. Please take my car. I am not allowed to drive it anyway." Eventually, I left her, thinking of Joseph, Tee Jay and Jo Jo. I wanted to be back.

Three hours later I parked her car in the hospital car park and reluctantly walked back to the ward. My heart sank as I walked past the office, seeing that two policemen were in there. I ignored everyone and walked to my room, only to be immediately summoned and escorted to the office. I stood in the doorway, reluctant to go in, and Alec sensed my difficulties. "Bridget, the car you were in was reported stolen to the police. Can you explain why you were driving it?"

I immediately felt sick again, as I was a law-abiding person in normal circumstances and I felt like a criminal. "Kim asked me to drive because she can't as she is on medication. I am not, and am allowed to drive other people's cars on my insurance." Both the policemen were looking at me. I felt myself blushing. One of them said, "We will need to see your driving licence and insurance." I nodded and turned to Alec, who was standing behind me blocking my exit to the doors. "I will have to ask Joseph to bring them in or take them to the police station." The policeman who had spoken nodded, and then I had to describe exactly where the bed and breakfast place was that we had booked. It appeared that Kim's fiancé had reported the car stolen. Afterwards, Alec asked one of the nurses to take me to my room. I sighed, as I knew I would again be labelled as trouble.

The next day Dr Lynn was in a serious mood. "Do you want us to help you or not? This is serious, Bridget. You need to work and I will help you, but if you don't want the help, there are plenty of other people who do and would appreciate it." I looked down at the floor, wishing it would swallow me up, but I also felt frustrated. "What about my dog? Doesn't anyone care? She is dead, and no one is bothered." Dr Lynn didn't answer; he just turned round on his way out. "By the way, you are now off level one as you showed some responsibility in coming back." His tall lean figure walked out of the door and down the corridor. I fell back on to my bed, feeling miserable and alone."

"See?" Sam said.

"See, what?" I shook my head, puzzled.

"See, people will want to read and know about that. I want to know if you found out who killed your dog and why." Sam suddenly went silent, as if she shouldn't have mentioned Jaz.

"Don't worry, I did find out and it wasn't straightforward." I sighed as it had taken me years to get over it, and I still wasn't sure I wanted to talk about it. "It was my mum. She had written 'do the necessary'." Sam looked shocked, but I continued.

"Mum was thinking about me and the kids. Jaz was dangerous and lethal, and I think Mum had the strength to do what I couldn't – I still wouldn't, even today. But I often think Jaz may have turned on someone. I don't know." Sam nodded and continued to watch the match. I thought back to the hospital, and although I was watching Tee Jay and the basketball, I reflected about hospital and my past.

People wouldn't understand about level ones and how they made you feel. First people tried to compare them as if it was happening to them. They didn't take into account the feelings of the patient. They didn't realise that the context and location had so much to do with it. Some days I hated the twenty-four-hour watch and accompaniment at close level, wanting my private space. I didn't want to have to think of limiting my drinks and watching what I ate because my toileting needs would be witnessed. I learned to plan ahead and to see which nurses would be on in the next shift so I could plan when to take a shower, who was the most lenient nurse, who would be satisfied with the toilet door just being ajar, or who would want to come and nearly sit on my knee. I learned to take all these factors into account. I also learned who could help me best when I was at my neediest, who would be the most fun nurse to go on a walk with, and which nurse was the best for me taking advantage of for sneaking a weapon into my room. I planned which shift I could do the most work with, or when to have visitors. I looked and observed, and sometimes I was so impulsive I scared myself. The hospital became a challenge, and the challenge took me to personal limits that I may not have reached had I been out.

***

Ward round always worked me up to the worst possible state, where I couldn't handle any change, good or bad. Ward round meant unpredictability. Ward round was a weekly event where 'the team' decided your future, your care and anything else they could think of. The team consisted of the team leader, who could be the consultant and the other people involved in your care, which could include social workers for some people as well as the medical staff. Ward round was supposed to be a chance for you to meet with your 'team' and for you to share your opinion and views with 'the team' on your care. It was a day that brought unrest to the ward, and if all this wasn't bad enough, on some weeks there were students invited to witness the patronisation of the unfortunate patient. This was just my personal view, and one that cannot be fairly backed up as I refused to attend ward rounds. Yet I had lived amongst others who had been in that situation and not once did I hear good feedback. I had been unfortunate enough to have been scolded and patronised right at the beginning by a nurse for not attending a ward round, and Dr Lynn had tried to bring some of his team into my room instead. The result was that I had panicked and tried to literally run through a wall. It was decided after that that I could be excused from the meetings. Although this helped in one way, as I was no longer panicking about having to attend, it also back-fired, as each time a ward round was held and the meeting was about me, I anticipated the worst. I did not trust who was in there. I paced up and down the corridor outside the room, worked up, frustrated and feeling completely out of control. The out-of-control feeling would escalate, and the anxiety would reach a pinnacle and I would act out impulsively without thinking. I would bolt for the window despite being a floor up, and I would try to smash my way through to the outside.

***

Flashback:
I bolted for the window, fist clenched, and hit out as hard as I could. I repeated this with strength and speed; the glass smashed, but the reinforced glue in between stopped the pieces falling to the ground. They clung, hanging in the air, while I leapt up onto the window sill, pushing my elbow and right leg through. Someone grabbed my left leg and I was pulled with force back into the room. I fell on top of a team of nurses, and I fought like a trapped animal to free myself from their grasp. They grabbed hold of any part of me they could cling onto, and my eyes swept the room for anything that I could grasp to hurt myself with. Someone pushed a mug out of my reach, and I was pushed onto the bed. I was panting and shaking, and I still forced myself up, nearly throwing two of them off. I could see the window and the opening and it drew me like a magnet. As four of them held me, another nurse started to examine my arms: I had a few minor cuts around my wrist where my fist had smashed through the glass, but apart from that I was fine. I sat and calmed down. The other nurses were sent out and Ruth glanced at me. "OK?" she asked. I nodded, taking a deep breath.
"Right, let's get you out of here until this is boarded up." I was escorted to the nurse's office and she beckoned me to sit down. "Tea or coffee?"
"Tea, thanks," I said, and sat back, exhausted.
"Can I trust you to sit there?" Ruth asked. I nodded and just stared at the floor and waited for a drink to be brought to me. It was, but in a plastic mug.
"What was all that about?" Ruth asked.
I shook my head. I didn't know myself. All I knew was that the panic came and I needed to get out.

***

The basketball game had finished, and we had won easily. We were in a good mood as we left the building. I went to offer Sam a lift back, and as I asked her if she wanted a lift, I suddenly remembered her saying that Tom's friend had thrown up all the way to Nottingham, and she had felt sorry for the person taking her. "Oh, I just remembered," I said, and she laughed, replying, "I was just going to remind you."

"Ha ha, do you know? Anyone else, I would have thought , shit, and wished I hadn't offered. You are a true friend and I am going to tell you forget about the lift, as I don't want that." She set off laughing as I collected Tee Jay and waved to her as she gained a lift back with the person who had taken her. On the way back in the car, I laughed as I related to Tee Jay what had happened. He was horrified.

"Mum, you can't do that."

"Why not?" I asked.

"Because Sam's your friend, and you can't let friends down." Tee Jay looked serious.

"I wasn't letting Sam down. She already had a lift, and I was being honest – that's what friends are for: to be honest with. And she didn't want me to give them a lift." I drove back, still laughing as I knew Sam would be laughing too. She was, as I asked her the next Saturday if her son's friend had thrown up again. I did give her and Tom and his friend a lift that Saturday, but it was only 100 yards down the road.

CHAPTER FIVE – JIGSAWS

I was invited to an event by the People's Forum to talk about my book, and I would be lying if I said I wasn't nervous. They had been very good to me and helped promote my book at one of their earlier events. I felt I owed it to them to turn up, and I also wanted to know what one of their events was like. I was a chicken, and I asked Sam if she would go with me. It would be the first event that I would have attended with Sam that didn't include watching our children play sport. Sam told me she would have to arrange it with her work but was pretty sure she could make the time off. I so hoped that she would like going and we would have a good time together.

Joseph had been skiing for a week in St Anton with the regular group of lads he went with previously. One of the men was our neighbour Martin, who was the husband of my good friend Joanie. They had a lot to celebrate when he was away, as his daughter Claire gave birth to his first grandchild. She had a little daughter, who she called Maisie. The men subsequently had to wet the baby's head.

A few weeks before, Joseph had travelled to Switzerland to see his parents. It was the first time since we had been married that he had gone on his own, as he always insisted we should go as a family. This time, though, he had some financial business to sort out with his parents, and I persuaded him to stay over for a week. Whilst he was gone, Jo Jo, Tee Jay and I had decided to give the playroom a makeover, and we also had some help from Paula, who was a very good friend of ours who first met us through Homestart, a charity that helped families.

"Mum, which brush do we use?" Tee Jay asked as he and Jo Jo started to pour the paint into the trays. I pointed out the correct brush and laughed as I watched their first attempt to cover the walls. It took us three coats, despite the "one coat" claim on the paint pot, and by the third coat I was happy. Tee Jay helped me lay the one-click laminate the next day whilst Jo Jo helped hang the curtains up. "I love this room now," Jo Jo stated as she tied the curtain back. I smiled as I surveyed the room. I was proud of my kids and couldn't wait to show Joseph when he got back.

When Joseph arrived back the kids showed him through to the playroom and waited with baited breath. "Fantastic!" he said, grinning at them both. "Who thought of the colour scheme?" "Mummy," they both said, looking at me. I smiled and waved my arms, gesturing at the curtains – cream in background with chocolate-covered squares, and the chocolate beanbags. "I did ask Jo Jo and Tee Jay first. It was mutual agreement."

I had been brought up with animals, and all animals that were introduced into our family became part of the family. We had names for every animal. The only exception was the fish tank, where some of the residents were named and others were not. Tee Jay was known as "chicken boy" to our friends, as he loved the poultry. He was in charge of our paddock, which housed chickens, ducks, quail, rabbits, guinea pigs and our four rescued billy goats. Tee Jay had insisted on rescuing two of the goats as a tenth birthday present, so whilst his friends asked for game boxes and bikes, all Tee Jay wanted was to rescue Brownie and Cadbury. He adored white chocolate at the time, and Brownie was a brown goat, whereas Cadbury was a plain white goat.

Jo Jo was a typical teenager with a typical teenage attitude. I was forever reminding her that our home was a home, not a hotel. I had long given up choosing clothes for her, as she was fashion-conscious, and I understood how important clothing was to her identity and status amongst her friends. There were still boundaries, though, and the clothes she chose first had to meet with my approval. Jo Jo was still a good kid, and she helped when I really insisted, and she was careful with her spending money. Jo Jo was lucky: she was brilliant at sport and very competitive, and she was fortunate to be clever and was in the top set for most subjects. Tee Jay was not so lucky. He had been diagnosed with specific learning difficulties, and had dyslexia. I had fought long and hard through his primary school years to access the support he required. I, with Joseph's support, battled to gain a special education needs statement. We were lucky that after we self-referred to an educational psychologist, we had the support of a brilliant senior psychologist who knew the ropes, and she battled with us to achieve a SEN statement for Tee Jay. We were worried he would still be teased at the next school. It turned out better than we had anticipated, as within days Tee Jay had made many new friends – most of them were girls, to our amusement, although he made new friends with some boys. He was also popular with the teachers, so although not as academic as Jo Jo, Tee Jay made up for it socially. Both children were proud that their mum had written a book, and they were proud of their dad, who was a professional wine consultant and recognised as one of the best in the world. They thought it was funny that Joseph had also appeared on television in a series on Channel Four that was called *Here's One I Made Earlier*. Now Tee Jay kept telling his friends' parents that his mum's book was number one in several categories. I wondered sadly whether he would still be as proud when he was grown up and understood the situation better.

***

I sat on the settee, trying to show Tee Jay how to use his BlackBerry. He had begged for one for Christmas, but after buying him one, I wasn't sure if I had done the right thing. He was now downloading games, and as his BlackBerry was getting fuller my pocket was feeling lighter. I felt that nowadays there was a lot more pressure on parents from their children to keep up with the rest of their friends. As I sat on the settee with the children, Joseph walked in from playing tennis at the local club. He thanked me for the dinner waiting for him in the oven. I laughed with Jo Jo; we declined to tell him that it had been intended for Tee Jay who at the last minute refused it as he had already eaten at his girlfriend's house. I would normally have cooked Joseph a dinner, but he had not been sure of what time he would be back, so earlier on I had told him to get his own. It had started to rain whilst we were watching the television, and suddenly I had a flashback to when I was younger before the hospital days and slept out rough.

***

Flashback:

It was pouring down, and I walked along the pavement, unsure where I was going or what I was going to do. I was tired, and my thoughts swung erratically in my head. My trainers were held together by the laces, and every now and again I felt the wet seep through from the sole. The bright lights of the cars dazzled my eyes, and I kept my head low, focusing on the pavement and the ground. I walked a few miles, heading towards Leicester, and it was to my relief that the dazzling brightness of the headlights became less frequent. It was getting on, and most people were in bed. I was now shuffling, and I dragged one foot after the other. I had lost track of time, and all I wanted to do was to lie down. As I walked along a hedgerow, a sudden gap in it became an invitation to be able to rest. The next field was empty, and I climbed wearily over the stile to cross it to make myself a place to lie down, sheltered from the rain. A low gap in the hedge further along was the best I could find. I sat huddled, trying desperately to put the longest bit of my coat under my thigh to stop the wet coming through. My hood shielded my face, and I lay down, my head resting on my arm. I was tired but my heart was beating rapidly, and I was conscious of the odd car driving on the opposite side, and I just hoped I would not be spotted. I eventually drifted off and woke to feel a scrambling across my hood. It was a rat, and I realised there were drains on the other side of the hedge. I didn't mind the wet, the isolation or the cold, but I could not put up with the rats and I wearily lifted myself to walk on.

***

39

Jo Jo's laughter brought me back to the television, and as the rain pelted on the window, I smiled to myself. I was indoors and safe with my children and husband around me. I tried to reflect why I was in such a state when I was younger. I knew I was on valium at the time, as I had suffered massive headaches from a major incident in Belgium, when I ashamedly had gone head first down a flight of steps. I had been in a state then, as I had been waiting for months for my biological mum to contact me, and she hadn't. It was at the time when I had suffered severe sexual abuse from several different people: the policeman, vet and bank manager, and of course Sandra. I had stayed with my relations in Belgium with Denny, and had enjoyed it so much I couldn't face going home. At the time I hadn't thought things through and had acted out impulsively. People would ask why I didn't tell people who loved me about my situation. The answer is that I was not fully aware of it myself. I was in despair, but didn't know why, and the suppressed feelings kept reasoning at bay and the denial was strong and at a forefront. All I could think about was that I had so wanted my biological mother to ring. I didn't even realise that anything was wrong. It was like a jigsaw: separate pieces pulled me apart and I acted out on pieces. At that stage, the pieces were not joined, and irrationality and impulsiveness took over. The end picture could not be seen, and it was as if my self-identity was in limbo, with only pieces acting out at separate times, so my real self was not intact. I can now look back a little and think that the longing I had to meet my real biological mother had been pulled out of perspective, as it was like a lifeline that would answer all my problems, although again I did not realise it at the time. I looked around at my family and wondered if I would ever be able to piece my jigsaw back together.

***

The next day dawned bright and sunny. I shouted upstairs. "Tee, hurry up, it's nearly nine o'clock and the hens need letting out." Five minutes later I could hear him moving around. He trundled downstairs and gave me a kiss as he poured himself some orange juice. "We need to move the electric fence, Mum," he said as he poured his cereal out. "I know. Hurry up, then." I smiled across at him and we rushed to get into the paddock. We started to move the fence and were in luck because the ground was soft and wet from the week of rain. But our luck didn't last, and by half ten it started to rain again, and it was also getting very cold. We had let Goldie and Leah out, our Sebastopol Frizzles – a rare breed of goose. They were bright white and looked like they had a ballerina skirt on. In the sun they looked beautiful, in the wet and mud, not so beautiful. "Mum!" Tee Jay shouted. I looked up, and he was filling the water butts up and wanted the water switching off. "Hurry up!" he shouted. I looked across at him to tell him off; I was no spring chicken and to climb over the netting wasn't as easy as it used to be, especially in wellies and deep mud. "Ha ha, very funny," I retorted. He was laughing like mad, hands on hips. Tee Jay had a great sense of humour just like Joseph, and Joseph's dad who we called Papi. I rushed, putting my hands out to stop Amba and Asti jumping up at me with their muddy paws, and turned the tap off. I returned back through the little gate to the paddock that stopped the dogs entering. Although I loved the dogs, they would both kill the poultry and attack the goats at the earliest chance possible. When we first had the poultry, I had to teach the cats very quickly to stop them chasing the hens. I only had to do it once with our eldest cat Petrus, yet both Siamese/Birman-cross cats Truffles and Cream would still chase and it was only after two or three shoutings, which I did each time as soon as they tried to jump on a hen, that they stopped chasing the hens. I hoped that Bella, our new kitten, would not chase them. She was very sweet: a pretty calico kitten with ginger, black and white markings. Tee Jay and I changed our 50-metre fence to try to make some separate areas, as we had a few trios and pairs of hens that needed to be kept apart. We were not in luck. The rain poured and we made a mess of it, as we forgot that once sealed off we could not cross through the fencing with the other fence. It was cold, and it was getting on for lunchtime. "Come on," I said to Tee Jay. "Forget it. We will do it when the sun is out, not when it is freezing." He nodded, little droplets of water falling off his fringe and running down his nose. I looked at him in his green wellies and khaki camouflage pair of overalls. He was growing up to be a young man, and he was quite mature for his age when it came to looking after his poultry. His dark brown eyes were huge, and with the thick long eyelashes coating them and dark complexion, he was very popular with the ladies as well as the girls. "Go ahead, Mum!" he shouted. "I'll finish off. I haven't much to do, and I will put Goldie and Leah back in." I stamped my feet to get the mud off my wellies and headed indoors. I left my boots outside under cover and hung my wax jacket on the peg and walked into the kitchen. Joseph had just finished cleaning and hoovering and was starting dinner. I smiled at him as I made my way to the shower room. I shouted up to Jo Jo, "Is Bella up there with you?"

"Yes," came back the answer. I washed my hands in the sink and went to check the emails on my computer. I checked on my book, *A Fine Line,* and it was still number one in child abuse. I read about the competition: the third book was a book about an abandoned child and its title, *Cut,* made me shiver.

***

CHAPTER SIX – RAZORS AND CIGARETTE LIGHTERS

The first time I cut was when I was still at school, and to be honest I can't remember my exact age. I can remember the occasion as if it was yesterday, though: I was in our family bathroom at home. I had gone to the toilet and was in the process of washing my hands when I caught sight of my dad's razor.

***

Flashback:
It was a good, solid razor made of gold-coloured metal. I picked it up and held it in my hand. I fingered it, feeling the smoothness of the metal, staring at the glistening of the little edge of blade that could be just seen. It was heavy in my hand, and I placed it onto the edge of the bath. I rolled my jeans up and placed my foot on top of the closed toilet lid. I picked up the razor and held it against my leg to the side of my calf and pulled it sideways. Almost immediately a trickle of blood started to run down my leg. I grabbed a piece of toilet roll and dabbed at it. I held the white tissue and stared at the bright red blood stains. It fascinated me and I quickly pulled the razor against my leg again. This time a bigger drop of blood appeared. I stared at the dark blob, and when it started to trickle it got lighter and lighter. I started to experiment, pressing harder or softer with the razor, each time stopping the blood trickling onto my white socks with the tissue. I changed direction on my leg and I kept to the same area. After around ten times, I stopped. I felt strange; I hadn't felt anything. I carefully wiped my dad's razor clean and put it exactly where I had found it. I pulled my sock up over one of the cuts and used a wad of toilet tissue to stop the blood touching my sock. The rest of the cuts had stopped bleeding and I pulled my jeans leg down over the cuts, flushed the tissue away and went out of the bathroom.

***

Tee Jay had come to sit beside me on the settee. He was looking up the Latin name for chicken for his homework, and I explained it was *gallus domesticus* and that *gallus* meant 'comb' in English. He yawned and started to write, peeping every now and again at the Scotland versus Ireland Six Nations rugby game. The sun started to shine, and I thought that we should have gone out to finish the fencing, then was too tired to get up and do it.

***

I stopped Tee Jay from reading what I was writing, as I didn't want him to know his mum used to cut. I was ashamed of it, although I didn't blame myself, as at the time it was the answer to my needs. I didn't understand why, as I didn't plan to go into the bathroom to look for the razor. I didn't plan to cut either – it sounds daft, but it just happened. Although once I had cut, I became addicted, and I wanted to cut again. Yet again this is inexplicable, as it was only when I was so distressed, and by distressed I don't mean tearful or crying, as I never felt like that. The feelings or thoughts I had made me want to cut, but what feelings or thoughts would make anyone want to cut? I asked myself that too, and I realised that it was the same routine ones that would be as regular to me as eating or drinking. I would feel an intensity of panic or despair that was worse than anyone's worst nightmare. Usually with a nightmare you wake up and it stops or eventually goes away. These feelings were so intense that you wanted to go to extreme measures for them to stop. These extreme measures could take all sorts of forms: they were usually termed as self-harm or suicidal thoughts. The biggest misinterpretation would also happen here, because as soon as 'suicidal' is mentioned, people think that the suicidal person is so depressed they want to die. My interpretation is that I would all of a sudden suffer from such intensity that I need to act out for it to stop, and some of the actions could be so extreme that they were suicidal. But this wasn't because I wanted to kill myself – far from it. I just wanted the thoughts that were so intense and intrusive to stop.

***

When I was in hospital the therapy was quite intense, and also it brought my past to the forefront. My past still didn't seem a big deal to me. If I tried to sum it up, it was about a period of time from when I was twelve years old to when I was in my thirties that was of continual extreme sexual abuse. It lasted for over twenty years, and included knifing, burning, rape, blackmail, physical and mental abuse, a couple of murder attempts and mixed in between all of this was a lot of love, hugs and what I thought of at the time as normality. The normality existed to such an extent that even my own family and closest of friends had no idea what was going on. My dad died years later, never knowing the full extent of my past. In hospital Dr Lynn had first asked me to draw a lifeline and to first fill in the significant dates. My main

43

way to express the past was to draw, and I would draw picture after picture. The majority of these would contain 'The Black'.

Sometimes the nurses, Dr Lynn, or Andrea (my community psychiatric nurse at the time) would ask about the meaning of the illustrations. This could then lead to me unintentionally acting out.

***

```
Flashback:
I  stared  at  the  paper.  I  had  drawn  a  symbolic
representation:  a  huge  black  cloud  covered  most  of  the
picture,  and  amongst  the  smudges  small  pair  of  feet  were
drawn  coming  out  of  the  cloud,.  They  could  only  be
partially  seen,  as  a  stronger  drawing  of  a  bigger  pair  of
feet  and  legs  were  drawn  over  them.  It  must  have  been
pretty  obvious  what  it  meant,  but  Andrea  asked  a
question.  "Whose  feet…?"  She  didn't  get  chance  to  finish,
as  I  bolted  off  the  bed  and  aimed  for  the  door.  Andrea
made  a  grab  for  me  and  I  just  pushed  with  all  my  strength
for  the  opening.  I  wasn't  thinking  straight,  and  I  ran
through  the  nearest  doors,  which  led  to  the  dormitory
opposite,  and  I  headed  for  the  window.  I  hit  it  hard  and
repeatedly  with  my  clenched  fist,  and  felt  the  crunch  of
the  pane  breaking.  Andrea  grabbed  my  left  arm,  but  my
right  arm  had  successfully  broken  through  and  I  could  see
my  freedom.  I  would  have  leapt,  but  the  tags  had  been
pulled  and  already  a  crowd  of  nurses  were  pulling  at  me
from  all  angles.  I  ended  up  on  the  floor,  panting  and
shaking.  I  caught  sight  of  a  mug  on  the  bedside  table  and
sprang  into  the  air  to  get  it,  but  someone  knocked  it  out
of  my  hand  and  Andrea  shouted,  "Hold  her!".
They  led  me  back  to  my  room,  and  I  was  pushed  gently
but  firmly  onto  my  bed.  The  drawing  was  still  visible,
and  Andrea  picked  it  up  and  gave  it  to  the  nurse  to  take
away.
  I  stared  at  Andrea.  She  was  older  than  me  and  I  guess
in  her  forties.  She  was  an  attractive  lady  with  a  big
smile  and  a  warm-hearted  grin.  She  made  me  smile  with  her
big  earrings  and  her  trendy  clothes.  I  liked  Andrea,  and
this  helped  a  lot  whilst  working  with  her  on  my  therapy.
The  pictures  I  drew  varied:  some  days  they  would  have
pictures  of  ropes,  razor  blades  and  the  cigarette  lighter
from  the  car.  Most  cars  had  these  cigarette  lighters
built  in,  usually  under  the  dashboard,  and  would  consist
of  a  mini-plunger  that  had  wire  elements  that  would  heat
up  at  the  end  when  the  cigarette  lighter  was  pushed  in.
When  the  device  was  pulled  out  you  could  see  the  red
wires  glowing  in  coils  at  one  end,  and  once  a  cigarette
was  pushed  against  it,  the  cigarette  would  light.  It
reminded  me  of  a  branding  iron  for  cattle.  I  remembered
```

what the bank manager would do when he held me down,
trapped in his car.

***

His car was white – a coincidence, as Sandra's car had
been white too. It smelt of cigarette smoke when you
first got in, but as always after some time in the seat,
I couldn't smell anything, feel anything, and at times
the closest I could think of the experience was to being
spaced out. The bank manager was the man who had asked me
to stay behind at the bank where I had worked, and
promised to help me find my biological mum. He had
invited a local counsellor to come and chat to me, and
had let me use the office address for her to give me
certain information. It was one day after the bank had
closed that he had asked me to stay behind so he could
help me further with finding my mum from the details the
counsellor had given me. I had stayed behind, and at the
young age of seventeen years old was probably a bit
naïve, but I genuinely thought he was going to help me.
He did help me with the information, but then brutally
threw me against some filing cabinets and raped me. This
was only the beginning, and as I had been groomed so
expertly by Sandra, I was in denial and suppressed most
of it. The incidents in the car are remembered in
fragments, and as with many of the episodes there are
complete blanks. Sometimes if the whole of an episode was
remembered, the times before and after are not
remembered. I could remember in detail when he would give
me a hug and comfort me, and it was these times that
remained in my mind.

***

I got into the car to take Jo Jo to a basketball match in Nottingham at the
Wild Cats Arena, where she played for a Melton team. It was foggy and wet,
and I was not looking forward to the journey as Joseph usually drove, but this
week he was in Geneva. Tee Jay asked if he could charge his iPod, and as I
pulled the cigarette lighter out to put the charger in I suffered a flashback.

***

Flashback:
The coils were bright red as he brought it close to my
skin. I could not protect myself as he had pulled any
clothing left off my body. I stared way past it, out
through the windscreen into the sky. His laughter echoed
around the car, and I still stared out into the sky. I
thought I could smell burning – that awful smell when you
accidentally singe your hair. I did it once when I
flicked Sandra's lighter for her. The flame had been high
and had caught my eyebrows, but now it wasn't my eyebrows

45

that had been burnt. The laughter echoed louder and I could hear my name being called.

***

CHAPTER SEVEN – DIABETES AND DINOSAURS

I turned around. Jo Jo was asking if I had remembered her drink. I nodded. "Look in the bag." Tee Jay passed her the bag and I started to reverse out of the drive. I headed for Nottingham and hoped I wouldn't get lost. The sat nav was my rescuer; the only time it let me down was when I had to change lanes quickly with no warning. Tonight Jo Jo was the only girl playing, and I laughed as the kit was big and her shorts were more like three-quarters. The Melton team played well and won by a point. We returned in a jovial mood, and Tee Jay ran through to let Bella the kitten out of the shower room. We had decided to call at the fish 'n' chip shop on the way back – a rare treat as fish and chips were not Joseph's favourite. It was great for me, as I hadn't eaten them for years, and it was nice to see the kids tucking in and licking their fingers. We sat laughing on the settee, joking about what Joseph would think. The time ticked by to ten o'clock, and I reluctantly told the kids they had to go to bed. It was a Friday night, but they both had basketball training in the morning, and both Jo Jo and Tee Jay put basketball before anything else. I checked the doors were locked and put Truffles and Cream into the corridor between the garage and the kitchen. Here they had a comfortable basket and access to the garden. Ginger and Petrus were allowed to stay in, as both were house-trained, although in the better weather they preferred to be out. The dogs stopped in the kitchen when the weather was bad; otherwise they liked to be in the garden where they had a big cosy kennel.

The next morning dawned bright and sunny, and I crept downstairs trying to keep quiet so that the kids could have another hour in bed. As I switched the kettle on I could hear the tapping of the woodpecker in the little spinney opposite the front of the house. I had used my new binoculars the week before and had caught sight of him in the neighbours' drive. The distinctive knocking was easier to trace than trying to sight him. He was a lesser-spotted woodpecker, and had returned to the area for many years. He had distinctive colours of black and white, with a flash of red on his head. He had driven me mad in the last couple of months, as I could always hear him and not see him, especially when I was in the paddock with the animals. Mum had given me some money for my birthday in January, and I had used it to buy a decent pair of binoculars. Now, as I could hear the knocking, I was more relaxed as I knew I had seen him. I let the cats in and made myself a cup of tea. It didn't taste half as nice now that I couldn't have sugar, so I sipped it reluctantly as I still couldn't face coffee first thing in the morning.

I had already taken a blood count for my sugar levels, and knew I had to eat pretty soon. I drank my tea and watched the news. When I was initially diagnosed with diabetes it came as a shock. I had been feeling really thirsty and had lost weight; also my eyesight had deteriorated suddenly. My doctor did a blood test and rang me the next morning to tell me the count was 19 and that diabetes was diagnosed at 11. I felt miserable, yet in one way relieved to have an answer. Although I hated the injections, I preferred the ones in the stomach to my thigh as they didn't usually hurt so much. I preferred the insulin, as it was more flexible, and if I wanted to eat extra or have the odd drink I could alter the dosage to my needs. I was not a good patient at first, and purposely took my body to the limits in defiance, thinking I could manage without. Of course I couldn't, and I learned the hard way. My first hypo – and I always got hyper and hypo mixed up, so I think it was hypo – was when I had just started to take my insulin.

***

Joseph had told us that we had to visit the Swiss Embassy in London to get the children's Swiss passports renewed. It was a subject that touched nerves, as when we went on holiday we always had an argument. I always booked with our British passports, which I was extremely proud of, and Joseph would always use the Swiss ones. I was glad that the children could have dual nationality, and I also had a Swiss passport, yet I was loyal to Britain first. Joseph felt different, as he had a Swiss passport and was loyal to his birth country. I could understand that, and most of the time there were no issues. We had fun when Wimbledon was on or when the world football took place, as we each teased the other.

Today we were up early, and for March the weather was lovely although still cold. Mick, our friend, took us to the railway station at Market Harborough where we found train tickets to London to be a lot cheaper than the Leicester run. The children were excited as it was a day off school, and they were also looking forward to the train journey. We had asked them where they wanted to go in London. Neither could make their minds up: Jo Jo wanted to go shopping and wanted to visit Harrods, while Tee Jay wanted to go to the Natural History Museum. I just wanted us to have quality family time. Jo Jo and I sat opposite Joseph and Tee Jay. The train was already packed and a noisy group of teenagers with tennis racquets kept most of the travellers' attention. The children couldn't get over the close proximity of another train travelling in the opposite direction, and twice Tee Jay jumped and we all started laughing. He and Joseph played cards, and Jo Jo read her book lounging against me. I tried to read, but couldn't concentrate and lazily watched the kids, and I kept looking at the chap in the opposite booth. He was reading with a device and I was fascinated. I couldn't make up my mind whether it was the new apple iPod or some sort of Kindle or other e-reader. It was the first I had seen, and I really wanted to get up and climb in the booth behind and look over his shoulder. I didn't.

We soon arrived in London and walked to the Swiss embassy. A man stood at the doors and we were not allowed in until we had confirmed our appointment and shown identity. We walked quietly through, and the atmosphere was like being in a library where you didn't dare sneeze and every noise was amplified. We were shown to a place that looked like a post office, where a lady sat behind a glass screen. Joseph passed the old passports under the glass towards her. She scrutinised each one carefully, and both children tried hard not to laugh as she stared at them with a very serious look. Tee Jay couldn't hold it in and burst out laughing, which made Jo Jo laugh too. Joseph looked uncomfortable and glared at him. We were OK: the lady smiled and asked Tee Jay his name. He was asked to sit in a camera booth and had a photograph taken. He then had to sign his name with some electronic equipment. Afterwards Jo Jo had to do the same and once the lady had all the details we were free to leave. We stepped into the sunshine, feeling relieved to be out.

"Where now?" asked Tee Jay, skipping, reminding me of Billy Elliot. Jo Jo walked up to me.

"Can we get something to eat, Mum?" I looked across at Joseph. I was a bit worried as I had taken my insulin, and it only being the first week wasn't sure if I needed anything. I had eaten a digestive biscuit earlier. "Let's have a walk first and look for somewhere on the way," suggested Joseph, already walking in one direction. The three of us skipped and walked to keep up with him, and we crossed the road to walk in the sunshine and not in the shade. We crossed by Marble Arch onto Hyde Park Corner, and then decided to walk across St James Park. It was a glorious day: the sun shone brightly and the bright yellow daffodils moved gently with the breeze. A grey squirrel darted amongst the tourists and stopped at a dropped ice cream cone.

We went on the Underground, and I grabbed hold of both the kids on the Tube as it was quite frightening how the doors opened automatically and shut. Jo Jo hovered near me and I could tell she was nervous. Tee Jay was busy looking at the route with Joseph, and they worked out we needed to get off at Embankment and walk towards London Bridge. I didn't know London that well, but we covered so much: we went to a little Italian restaurant, and it was there that I made a vital mistake with my diet. Normally I would choose chips and anything with chips, but due to my new instructions I chose a healthy salmon salad. We were not served any bread, and I declined a pudding, thinking I was eating healthily. Afterwards we walked to Harrods and toured the store. It was nice but very tiring, and after Jo Jo was satisfied she had seen what she wanted, we left the store to head to the Natural History Museum. It was a long trek, but the sun was out and we were all quite joyful.

Tee Jay loved dinosaurs, and couldn't wait to see them. We eventually entered the building and headed for the dinosaurs, and we started to walk up a metal stairway onto a ramp to look at the triceratops skeleton. It was whilst I was staring at the skeleton that I suddenly felt ill, and it came on so fast. I started to sweat, and I turned to Jo Jo. It was very dark, so I could hardly see her. It was alarming, as I was on a ramp high off the ground. "Are you hot?" I asked. She nodded and walked on towards Joseph. He was moving on and by now my legs felt shaky and I had a job to catch up. "Joseph, I have to stop and do a blood check." He walked on, and I felt so ill that I was sweating a lot and my top was wet through. "Joseph," I pulled desperately at his sleeve.

"I can't do anything now, can I?" he retorted and turned back to the dinosaurs. I looked for Jo Jo. "I need to sit down." She looked worried. "Let's try down there. Come on, Mum." I followed her down the ramp, hardly being able to stand, and we were in luck: there were two 3D virtual dinosaurs roaring and moving, but underneath was a silver metal visitor's bench. I nearly fell onto it. My strength was gone, and I had a job to prick my finger to take a blood count. I did manage and it was 3. I had been told not to let it fall below 4. I had some glucose lozenges in my bag, and took three at once. The kids were hovering anxiously and Joseph looked worried. I tried to play it down. "I'll be fine. Give me twenty minutes. You two go on and carry on looking around the corner." Tee Jay and Jo Jo ran round the corner and I sat back on my seat. I couldn't stand up, my heart was beating so fast, and I was still sweating. My legs were like jelly. Joseph got up to go, but I tugged his sleeve. "I want to, but I can't. You will have to wait for twenty minutes." He shrugged his shoulders, hands in his pockets, looking concerned.

A while later we headed for the café. Still weak, I ate a chocolate cookie and had a cup of tea. My blood count rose to 6.2. "I am OK to go," I said, fed up with looking at the stuffed panda that was opposite our table. We walked outside, past the Victoria and Albert Museum. Joseph decided we should walk across the park to Buckingham Palace. "I'll do my best," I said to him, "but I'm still a bit shaky." He held my hand and we walked slowly across the park and along the river. Everywhere I looked people were strolling in the sunshine. The daffodils brightened up the grass and the grey squirrels played. I decided that an ice cream wouldn't hurt, as I had a low sugar count, and I enjoyed being able to have one with the others. I realised my mistake in not eating enough carbohydrates at lunchtime. We sat on a bench enjoying the ice cream, and then we headed for Buckingham Palace. "Look, Mum," Tee Jay grabbed my arm and pointed. I looked to where he pointed, and to the left of Buckingham Palace in the park by a river, way down below the bridge, a man with straggly long hair and a huge beard was washing his socks in the river. Tee Jay was more interested in him then seeing the palace. He went to take a photo and I stopped him. "No, you can't do that."

"Oh, why not?" He looked at me with puppy-dog eyes.

"It won't work." I pulled a face at him. "Come on, let's go over the road and see the 'Changing of the Guard.' Tee Jay pulled a face and we both hurried to catch up to Jo Jo and Joseph, who had already started to walk towards Buckingham Palace. The flag was up, so the Queen was in residence. Joseph kept teasing the children, saying she was at the window. We eventually caught a late train back, and arrived home tired but happy. I hadn't enjoyed being ill, but I had learned from the experience. I was slightly irritated that Joseph hadn't supported me at the time, but when he realised how it had affected me, he had responded, and thinking about it he had to learn about the illness, just like me.

***

It was March 2nd 2011, and the kids were at school and Joseph was at a funeral. I had just come in from dashing to the paddock, as the goats had been bleating loudly. It was Billy, one of the pygmy goats; he always went for the others and had decided to bully Cadbury again. Cadbury was looking very muddy, and I could see that Billy had butted him along the side of his body. I intervened and gave them all some hay and went to check on the rest of the poultry before coming in. I could hear the male budgerigars having squabbles (with each other,) a sign of spring when all the males that usually got on well started to argue and try to dominate. It amazed me that as I drove home from the school run there were daffodils out in the neighbouring estate, but as soon as you turned up the private lane leading to our house, there was not a burst of yellow in sight. We even had some very late snowdrops still out. It was only half a mile up the road to the bright yellow blooms I had just driven by.

I was busy for the school run as Jo Jo and Bethany came out at 3.45pm and then Tee Jay had a basketball practice and came out at 4.30pm. I took the girls home and then went and picked Tee Jay up. "Mum, Mum, we have a match tomorrow at Oadby. It is a county one and we represent Melton Mowbray. Can you come and watch?"

"What time?" I asked, already realising any plans I had would fall through.

"1.30pm until 5-5.50pm," he answered. I thought about it, and I would have a job to do anything else. "Is Sam going?" I asked. I still didn't like going to new places on my own, and I knew Tee Jay would be travelling with the school. "That's the other thing I have to tell you," Tee Jay explained. "I have a form for Tom. Can we call at their house on the way home?" Kids – they sure do land you in it. I wasn't sure if Sam would mind me turning up, as it was only a couple of days ago she had told me where she lived. "OK, I'll drop you off and turn the car around." I dropped Tee Jay outside Sam's house, which was two minutes in the car from our house. Unfortunately the road we came out on from our lane was too dangerous to walk along. By the time I had turned the car around, Sam was on the pavement waiting for me to turn up. She smiled and was dressed in a jogging suit. I was relieved to see her smile as she worked nights and I hadn't wanted to disturb her. "Do you want to go?" I asked. She nodded eagerly. "I'll ring the school and see if we can grab a lift again on the mini bus," she said.

"OK, text me in the morning or I'll ring you," I answered, and Tee Jay jumped into the car and we waved goodbye to Sam and Tom, who had come out to see us.

Later that evening Sam rang me. "It's at Fulhurst College," she said. "I asked about a lift but the teacher said he had to see because of the insurance."

I laughed and said, "Did you say we had both been numerous times on that bus?"

Sam said, "I know, I said that, but he is new so he said he would have to ask. I'll let you know when I find out."

"OK, I will look the place up so I know where we are going. I will either pick you up to go the school or pick you up to go straight to Fulhurst. Text me when you know, or ring."

"OK," replied Sam, and I put the phone back and went back into the lounge where Jo Jo was revising. Joseph sat with a glass of red wine and Tee Jay was following me through. The table was prepared and I took the lid off the casserole dish, which contained the spaghetti bolognese that I had recently made. Luckily it was still hot, and we all sat down to eat. After dinner I went onto my computer to Google-search the college. I received a shock when I saw where it was. It was in the area where I had worked in the bank many years ago, and as I read the familiar names of the roads, I felt panic and despair flood through me.

***

Flashback:
His hands gripped my wrists tightly and he pushed them hard to the ground. I could smell the stale scent of cigarettes as he laughed, forcing his mouth onto mine. He was on top of me and he fumbled beneath my skirt. I looked into the branches of the rose bush nearby. The thorns looked lethal, but not as lethal as him. I knew he had entered me and I could also see the shocked look on the face of the young woman walking her pram on the footpath. He laughed and called out to her, "Lovely day isn't it!". The scurry of her heels and the spinning of the pram wheels spelt out her reaction. My face was covered by his jacket, and I kept my head down. Ashamed, guilty, sick, were all words tossing about in my head. The truth was I felt nothing. He had lit a cigarette and was puffing the smoke in my face, laughing he turned over and rolled onto his back. I quickly pulled my skirt down and attempted to do the buttons up on my blouse. The sun went behind a cloud and I pulled my coat tight around me.

He lay on his side, arm bent at elbow, hand propping up his head. His thick blond hair and steely blue eyes made him look years younger than he really was. "Nice park, this, isn't it?" he said. He had a habit of ending his sentences with 'isn't it'. I looked around. It could have been a million miles away; I didn't feel I was sitting in a park. I wasn't even sure if I existed. I guessed I did, as I think it was me sitting there next to that man. It was a weird feeling: I could see myself, a young dark-haired girl, sitting on the floor pulling my coat closely around me just staring out into space. There was a man there; he was wearing his grey suit as usual, with a cigarette packet just edging out of the top pocket. His lighter was a gold flat oblong one that flicked and a spark lit the gas. He was combing his hair and he suddenly jumped up. "Right, I am off. Be back within twenty minutes."

Fifteen minutes later I had walked the quarter of a mile back along the road to the bank. As I pushed open the doors, Mrs Coleman was walking out. I smiled. She was one of my favourite customers. I rang the bell, yet already he was there, opening the door to the staff side of the bank to let me in. "Hello, I hope you had a nice time out there in the glorious weather." He laughed and I pushed by him to put my coat on the hook. By the time I had reached my chair at the till, he had disappeared into his office.

***

Many people asked why Bridget let it happen time and time again. I have a job to explain even now, as it seemed like a dream, and it was as if I was watching it or remembering it as someone else. At the time the events were so pushed back in my mind it was as if they had never happened and when they did it wasn't real. If there had been just one person who had noticed something was wrong or someone had cared enough to notice, intervention might have helped. I feel upset that my mum hadn't helped. She had noticed the cuts and self-harm, even though Bridget had kept long sleeved cardigans on throughout the summer. My mum told me that her friend who had been a nurse had told her to ignore it as I was attention-seeking. It couldn't have been further from the truth, as the cutting was done in private and most of the time was concealed. Bridget didn't even know what was going on, and was so much in denial that it wasn't as if she could have asked for help as the people who in her mind were helping her were her abusers.

***

We were lucky, as Tee Jay's school decided that there was extra room on the mini bus, and Sam, her eldest son Damon, and I were offered a ride to Fulhurst. We accepted gratefully, and at 1.45pm we were heading out of

Melton towards Leicester. The teacher who was driving was fairly new to the area, so I shouted instructions to him to get on the M1, which seemed the most direct route. It also cut out the area I dreaded the most. The team was in a jovial mood, and we laughed most of the way there. When we arrived there were several other school teams waiting. Our group seemed to be the loudest, the most excitable and motivated team at the event. We didn't know what to expect, and just knew that the other competing teams had all won their own area competition. As the boys waited and then warmed up on the inside basketball court, Sam chatted to me. "Look at that, we have no worries." She was laughing, yet as I watched the first round of the competition the two teams playing first didn't handle the ball that well and we both knew that for the first half of the draw our team should win. "I don't think we should take it for granted," I said to Sam as we now watched our sons playing; the initial teams had now got into their stride and were playing so much better. Sam nodded. "Come on!" we both shouted in unison as our school scored. We clapped and sat back. The first game was in the bag. We won the next one and were in the semis – this was close, and eventually we swung it our way as our lads scored basket after basket. It was in the final that for the first time we didn't relax. The opposing team was good – so good that they went into the lead and I could hardly bear to watch. Just with a few minutes left, the teacher decided to pull off Tom, who was one of the best players, and play a different boy. "What the hell does he think he is doing?" We both said it at the same time and burst out laughing, but it wasn't funny and the opposition went and scored three baskets on the trot. "I can't watch. I feel sick," I moaned.

"What's the score?" Sam asked.

"I don't know, but there isn't much in it," I answered. Just then Ed was fouled and we had two free shots. We both went silent, willing the ball to go in. Ed was a little lad, but he was such a good player and we watched as he steadied himself and threw the first. It landed clean through the net. He passed the ball to the referee, who passed it back to him. He steadied himself, checking his feet were planted firmly behind the line, bounced the ball a couple of times and then bent both his knees and thrust the basketball forward high into the air. It was a clean basket, and we clapped happily as he scored the full two baskets. The referee blew his whistle and both teams ran to the scoring desk, including the coaches as nobody was sure who had won. There was suddenly an ear-splitting roar and as I looked to see which team was jumping up and down, I smiled. Our lads had done it: we were walking away with the county title. The opposition hung their heads in disbelief. It had been a close call, and apparently they had two baskets taken off for an earlier mistake and our team had gained two from Ed's shots and we won by two. The lads were ecstatic and we smiled as their teacher came over. "Thank goodness for that. When I took Tom off I was so knowing my name would be mud if we lost," he said. Sam and I looked at each other, and then looked at him. "Yes," we both said together, and he laughed. The drive home was unforgettable, with the lads were singing *We are the Champions*, and the teacher had decided to go through Leicester as it was peak time, and we were now driving through the area I had dreaded most. I stared silently through the fogged up windows at the park railings as we drove by. It was over twenty years on, and nothing had changed – even the rose gardens were still there. I took a deep breath, as I knew that we were going to go past the bank – the bank where he had first raped me, the bank where he had tortured me in the safes, the bank where I had first found out about my biological mother, and the price I paid for it. The mini bus drove by, and I had to look: the building hadn't changed. It still stood on the corner, and the memories were still there. Sam stared at me anxiously. I looked at her and smiled. "I think I am supposed to feel something, yet I feel like I am on a spaceship and everything around me isn't real." She seemed to relax. I sat back, not even feeling my seat. It was such a weird feeling. I felt like I was floating and floating away in a bubble where nothing could touch me and I couldn't feel anything. Suddenly the bubble burst. "Can I get off here?" Sam asked. I looked at her, puzzled. "I was going to see my dad in hospital tonight, and this will save me catching a bus back into town," she explained. I nodded and understood straightaway. "Will this do here?" the teacher asked. He was pulling up into a bus stop and taxi area. Sam stood up and I undid my seatbelt so I could let her out from the seat. Her son Damon stood up too. He let his mum go past and then sat down again. "Feed the kids for me," Sam instructed him as she got off the bus. He nodded and I waved as we set off on our way back to Melton again. I watched Sam's slight figure crossing the road. She was a pretty girl, possibly mid-thirties as Damon was about eighteen years old. I guessed she was mixed race, as her skin was quite dark, yet I was no expert. All I knew was that she was quite pretty and tough and vulnerable all rolled together in one. We hadn't known each other that long, and I was looking forward to going to the People's Forum together the next day.

CHAPTER EIGHT – MEETINGS AND LODGES

I picked Sam up at just before half eight and dropped the kids off at school. Sam laughed as we headed towards town. "Are you nervous?" she asked. I nodded as I glanced at my mirror at the car behind. "You bet, but not as bad as I anticipated. I just hope we find it OK." Sam nodded and replied, "We will, as my ex-boyfriend lived in the same street. I know where it is."

I breathed a sigh of relief. We arrived there within half an hour and drove into a car park. We asked the car park attendance chap if there was a place reserved for us. He checked on a list and pointed us to a parking spot. "Thank you," I smiled at him and steered my vehicle into the place he pointed to. Sam jumped out of the car carrying a bright red shoulder bag. It already came in useful as we put some of my books into it. We entered the building; it was very grand and had been used as a masonic hall in the past. I signed in with Sam and introduced ourselves to the appropriate person. We were shown through to a large room where tea and coffee was being served. We both sat down with a cup of tea. I stared around the surroundings and my heart gave a little lurch as I realised that in all the years I was a child, all the times my dad was at London Road, it was in this building he came to. The place was decorated with big wooden shields representing the appropriate lodges. I racked my brains trying to remember which lodges my dad attended. I knew he had been a Grand Master at one of them, and even higher up at another. As I looked at all the names of the different lodges on the shields, I recognised the Roundhill Lodge as being a lodge my dad belonged to. "Sam, we must find the board and look, as my dad's name should be on there. It would be fantastic to see my dad's name on it." Sam was already off and peering up at some of the boards. We searched corridor after corridor, and then there it was towards the end, the board with Roundhill on it. I looked down the list of dates. I read my dad's name, listed against the year 1976. I felt really proud and felt a moment of closeness to him. I hoped he would be looking down at me and be proud of my book. Deep down I don't think he would have been proud, as he would not have liked the content. I questioned myself to as whether he would have been able to have seen the bigger picture, past the content and to see how the book would have been so beneficial for the insight it gave. I decided not. My dad was always a gentleman, and slightly Victorian in nature. I think he would have put his reputation first and denied the book existed. My dad was very British, stiff upper lip and all that went with it. I sighed and thought to myself, 'Well, Dad, they will be speaking about me soon and will you look down and smile or will you not?'. Ironic, I thought, that the speech about me and my writing achievements was in the very building that my dad spent a lot of time in.

It was a while later that we were all asked to sit down in front of the stage in the central building. I sat at the back, a little nervous about what was going to be said. In the end I need not have worried as the speech was pretty straightforward and quite factual about the book reaching number one in several categories, and they used my quotes of how I was no expert but there were ways and means around problems nowadays, and support there if you looked for it. Sam sat next to me and we both sat being slightly wary, apprehensive and quite focused.

After the speech several people asked me if they could talk to me later about writing a book. I was secretly bemused and felt privileged that people did want to ask my opinion. I sat down and had a cup of tea with Sam and we were immediately approached by an elderly man wanting to ask about writing his own book. Afterwards I attended an education workshop to chat about the Open University, and how it had opened the door for me to work on my psychology degree. I only had praise as the university had given me so much support and had taken all my disability needs into account. I had been allowed to take a home exam, receive telephone support and have the support of a learner support team when I suffered some setbacks relating to my personal circumstances.

My reward for chatting about the Open University was when a young man came up to me and told me that my talk had really inspired him. He came and chatted to me in the afternoon and told me he had always been interested in psychology. Sam later told me that he had told her he had attempted suicide earlier in the year, and it turned out that his father-in-law had died, and he was the person who had given him a lot of support in the past. He was a pleasant young man with a third child on the way, and I hoped that he managed to receive the support that was essentially needed. I came away with mixed feeling about The People's Forum, as although they represented a significant body to fight for mental health issues, I personally disliked the way the event took place. In my opinion the mental health users were completely segregated from the organisers. We were herded to the seats for the presentations whilst the organisers stayed at the back, and then people were clearly directed to different areas for the various events that had taken place. Sam had picked this up and mentioned it on the way home and I thought it was a shame as they also did a lot of good. I also appreciated the support they had given to my book, which they didn't have to do. Yet I also realised that the event must have taken a lot of organising and may have needed this routine to work. Also The People's Forum had supported me for my first book and I wondered if they helped others with their projects and aims. The event they had put on had been free and I think it must have motivated and supported some of the users there.

CHAPTER NINE – THE CHAIR

It was a Monday morning and I was on my way to the diabetic clinic to see Maggie. The car park was full at the surgery, so I parked at the local supermarket and walked across the road. I felt nervous and apprehensive, as I still hated to wait in any waiting room even when they were open plan. As I walked around the corner I was in luck: only the receptionist was there. I asked her to let Maggie know I had arrived and went to sit down. I usually sat at the end, but a chair with high arms had been placed at the end of the seating for people who had difficulty in getting up. I sat on the end of the seat next to it and opened my iPhone to see if I had any messages. All the time I was aware of anyone who came or went by. A young lad in military clothing sat down in the far corner and then an elderly man checked in and went and sat down next to the young man in the uniform. The elderly man introduced himself and started to tell the young chap that he had been in the army when he was younger. Another person came and sat down, and now I was really nervous. I hated to wait, and I didn't like to wait with people. It panicked me. I sat close to the empty chair next to me and all the time I was so hoping no one would come and occupy this chair. In the time I had been waiting I had become obsessed about the chair. This chair blocked my exit out and I leaned heavily on one of the arm rests, hoping that Maggie would appear and call me in. I did not want anyone to sit in this chair, and all I could think about was should I sit and wait? Should I walk out now? The seconds started to feel like minutes, and the minutes felt like hours. I switched my iPhone on; I switched my iPhone off. I watched and waited, and it was only a few seconds later that my worst scenario came true. An elderly man with a walking stick walked slowly up to the receptionist and checked himself in. I noted straightaway as he gave his name that he had looked at the chair – the chair that I was leaning on, the chair that was so important to keep free. It was like everything had gone into slow motion as he used his walking stick to lean on as he struggled to walk over to the chair. "Excuse me," he said, looking at me. "I need that chair." I had already grabbed my handbag and shuffled away from it, feeling guilty that I had been leaning on this chair. I looked to my left, and the next person sat quite a distance away so there was room for me to move a little, but already the elderly man had sat down and I froze…

***

Flashback:
He edged towards me and I pushed hard backwards. I was back in Belgium in my cousin's next-door neighbour's house. I was stuck between the kitchen table and the wall. I could not get out, as he had sat down and was now moving towards me. My hand reached out and my fingers scraped the wall. I was cornered, and as I sat there looking around his kitchen, he pushed a cold custard blancmange in front of me. The top of it was wrinkled and the skin rippled. He pushed a spoon towards me and spoke with a strong Walloon accent that was common in some parts of Belgium. I felt sick, and the sight of the blancmange dish repulsed me, yet it was nothing compared to the old man who was leering at me and edging towards me slowly yet determinedly. My back was already pushed into the corner, and I hurriedly reached for the spoon and dug the tip of it through the thick rippled skin that tore apart to reveal a yellow-beige mucus. I ate it because I dreaded the worst, and smiled falsely as the mixture slithered down my throat, trying hard not to choke on the lumps and the foul smell that was seeping through my nostrils. The stench was not from the blancmange; it was from my cousin's neighbour who had enticed me into his kitchen and who was now edging towards me in his dirty brown trousers, shirt and braces. He must have been in his eighties, but he was intent on moving nearer and nearer. He was laughing, and I could not understand his strong accent, yet his body language was speaking out clearly. In desperation I reached out for the blancmange to give myself time to think. I swallowed hard, and as my stomach heaved I put my hand over my mouth to stop myself throwing up. He laughed at this, and his hand grabbed my thigh in jest. It was to my relief that he suddenly started to eat his blancmange, and then he moved away from me to shuffle into his cold pantry to offer me another blancmange. It was in this second that I leapt up from my seat as if someone had released my coils. I only had a second and I took it. I muttered, 'Merci', and nearly ran from the room. He turned round, startled, with a blancmange in each hand. He placed them on the table quickly and started to approach me, clearly unhappy and speaking loudly and fast. I opened the door and once out I breathed the fresh

60

air deep into my lungs and ran to my cousin's house and let myself in, locked the door and went upstairs to my room. I looked out of the window, expecting him to come chasing round. He did not, but I kept the door locked for the rest of the morning.

***

I looked up. Maggie had come out of her room and was walking towards me. She was a petite lady, always smartly dressed and with a smile on her face. She made me laugh, as she was so professional yet sort of mischievous, and I guessed she would be a good match for anyone who would ever dare to cross her. I was glad she was my diabetic nurse, as she was quite caring, but would also be very honest and tell you off if you deserved it. It was nice to be able to chat to her as I had learned that even my moods could affect the stability of my diabetes and vice versa. This morning Maggie was quite cheerful but had immediately picked up on my sombre mood. "Ignore me," I said, and I flung my coat onto the opposite chair in her room. "I am a bit panicky as I had to wait, and I was trapped by that old man."

"Don't worry, we wouldn't let anything happen to you here," said Maggie. I smiled. It was hard to explain that the damage had already been done and that the distress had seeped through on the inside even if it could not be expelled to the outside. I had relived and re-experienced something that I didn't want to, and even in the past I had not really felt any emotions, and reliving it again I had felt numb, but the repulsiveness sort of lingered around. I could not explain it properly, but it was like being taken back to a bad nightmare that hadn't been released and remembering it and experiencing it and again not being able to release the emotions and just pushing it away. It meant that every time something familiar that would remind me of that event would bring it all back, I would be there living it. Maggie would see it as the elderly man in the chair in the waiting room being a threat to me as I was scared of him. I was not scared of him. It was the associations that his actions brought to me that was unpleasant. Maggie and all the staff in the world could not do anything about that. I smiled at her as she continued to say that I had made progress, as a few months back I would not have been able to sit in the waiting room, and she had to fetch me in from outside. I so wanted to try to tell her how much better that was, as it cut down the risk and associations of being trapped and feeling as repulsed as I did. I showed Maggie my diabetic record and she advised me on the adjustment for my insulin as it was still a trial and error: one week she would be telling me to increase the insulin and the next week I could be advised to cut it down. It was never straightforward or predictable, or even rational, as the readings did not always relate to the food and sugar levels. The causal relationship between food and readings was unfathomable, and I had given up on the logical side. I teased Maggie as I left, telling her I was going to mention her in my next book. I laughed as I shut the door on her bemused expression.

***

Maggie was just one of the recent people in my life who had restored my confidence in people a little bit. It was awkward, and due to my past – and I am not even sure if it is my past, as even in the present, relationships with people are still very Machiavellian. I could not take it at face value that anyone would wish to show kindness or help without there being a trade-off. Maggie seemed genuine, but in my past so had many other people who had all let me down in a big way.

I am not sure who I think let me down the most, and if I started to go through the people who had hurt and let me down then I would not have enough room in the book. As I write this, I realise I don't want to convey who they are, as life is very delicate and far too short. I also want to concentrate on the good things in my life. Yet I also understand that if I just accept that people do let you down and there is no hope for me to have friends, as they will do the same. Yet in my past many people did let me down, which then makes me ask the question: why? Was it my fault? Did I ask for it? Or is it that you just have to accept people do let you down, or was I just so unlucky? I want to have friends, and I would like to think that they would not let me down. How will I know, and do I take the risk? I am not paranoid or ill; I am going on experience from my past, and sadly my past teaches me not to trust people. I could also examine my past, and ask the question, "does everyone let everyone else down, and people around me accept that people do this and just move on?". This would then lead me on to the question of identifying how significant the meaning of 'let down' is. Once identified, does the word 'tolerance' come into play? If 'let down' just means someone forgot to telephone or meet someone, then I could be pretty tolerant of that. If 'let down' means that someone built your trust and then abused it, I would have to think about it. If 'let down' means that someone tried to rape you or burn you, then I would be wary of people. If 'let down' also means that someone befriended you and then tried to kill you, I would be wary of that too. If I went through the number of attempts when I was significantly harmed, then in my world it would be more surprising if I ever had a relationship or trusted any one person again.

I also found it quite patronising that because in my past I was severely abused, raped, survived several murder attempts and survived against the odds, that I was judged to have a mental health problem. The people who were all sick enough to do this to me continued to live their lives unscathed. I had a reason not to trust people, and it was a rational reason. I believe to this day that my everyday actions are a rational response when placed in context with my past. Yes, I have a job to stay in the same room as people, but then when you find out that for over twenty years I was continually locked up, raped and abused, then it makes sense that I would not be comfortable being in the same room as others. If my past had not happened and I was uncomfortable being amongst people then I would think I was mentally ill.

This is just one example of my life being upside down. Another example is that I genuinely get upset and wary if people are nice to me. I start to wonder what they are after, but again this makes sense when put into context with my past. Yet I am relaxed if people are rough, rude and possibly threatening, as this means they are showing their true colours and I know where I stand and what to expect. As I type this onto my laptop I am already thinking some readers will have a job to understand this and are classing me as ill, but I am just trying to explain. I try to look at it from all angles, and I can see that the average person would be more relaxed when someone was nice and feel threatened if someone was unpleasant. The average person would have been conditioned to accept these issues as normal. I had been conditioned to accept the opposite way round as normal. Whether I was ill or not depended on the context.

***

I was sitting on the settee next to Tee Jay watching *Masterchef*. It was nice to see Michel Roux Senior on the program, as I had met him and Joseph had known him for nearly thirty years. Michel Roux had also written a message in one of his cooking books to my mum, praising her apple pies; the book had been given to her as a Christmas present. Amba and Asti were lying on the blanket in the corner, and our five cats were scattered around the house. Joseph had gone to watch the television in bed and JoJo was on her laptop in her bedroom. I had been busy working on the paddock the last few days trying to get some organisation into our tiny smallholding. All my animals seemed to have problems: Pumpkin, my gander, ignored his female partner and preferred Tee Jay. He would get frisky and try to climb on Tee Jay, and my cockatiel had paired up with a budgerigar. We also had a cockerel called Little One who was brought up by a duck, who now only mounted the ducks even though he had plenty of hens around. My mum would laugh when she walked around our paddock, but apart from these incidents we still loved all of the animals, as they were quite cute. We had rabbits and guinea pigs, a chipmunk called Roland, some quails, hens and ducks, and we also had an aviary with the budgies and cockatiels. The goats lived at the bottom of the paddock, and Billy always bleated as soon as he heard us. Bella, my kitten, came running up and she made me laugh as she threw herself into the air after a fly. It was with my family and my animals that I found my peace, feeling no threat. I sometimes got stressed, as I worried about the care for both my family and animals. I was very sensitive and hoped that my family, including my animals, were well looked after most of the time. When I went on holiday, which was only once a year unless we visited Joseph's parents, I would worry about whether the animals were OK and be so glad once we got home and I had counted every single pet.

Today Sam was at our house and Tom was still learning to look after the hens. We had recently bought some point-of-lay chickens from a little smallholding on the borders of Warwickshire. We had bought four pied, one lavender, three coucou and four copper blacks, which Tee Jay still swore were black rocks.

The ladies had settled in well, and Tee Jay had named the coucous after the ladies at the local post office. It seemed funny when he was shouting, 'I have lost Little Margaret and can you catch Big Boss Margaret,' as I pictured the ladies at the post office not the hens he was talking about. They were amused and it was nice to have such a friendly atmosphere when we were at our local post office. They had all read my first book and they were all very fond of Tee Jay. Jane, one of the ladies, had actually asked her daughter and husband to take Tee Jay to a local Tiger's rugby match where he was spoilt and had the chance to meet Martin Castrogiovanni, the Italian player. Tee Jay also liked them a lot, and liked being teased by Debbie who had a son a year older than Tee Jay. It was by coincidence that Little Margaret had placed the closed sign up just as Tee Jay was in the queue, so they had a standing joke about the closed sign. He always said that one of the Margarets would buy the eggs when we had some spare, and he was right and Jane helped us out a lot too. Although the ladies at the post office were unaware, their friendship had helped me so much, and it was a big boost to my self-confidence that we could chat to them.

It was coming up to Easter and I had been decorating Tee Jay's room and trying to build his furniture. I had managed to build a three-door wardrobe and a chest of drawers. Today was Saturday, and I had got up early to start on the bed, which had drawers underneath. I was now in a bad mood as I had started at 8am and the weather was glorious, and it had gone past three o clock and we were still finishing the bed. The trouble was we had built it then Tee Jay had decided he wanted it in a different corner of his bedroom, which meant taking the bed to pieces again as the drawers opened to the wall instead of into the room. The other niggling factor was that the goose eggs, which were in an incubator in Tee Jay's room, had started to chip and a gosling was trying to hatch and every time I used the hammer I was aware of this little bird making an attempt of breaking through into our world. Here was I using a hammer so easily and here was a gosling that was so worn out after hammering away for twelve hours to come out of his shell. By evening time the remaining two eggs had also started to show signs of life. Tee Jay also came running back from the paddock to say that Leah, our Sebastopol Frizzle, had got goslings in her nest. We had also peeped into the budgie's nest box and had seen a blue fledgling and a green fledgling. We also laughed as the female mum, who was a white budgerigar, was landing on the quails' back and having a piggyback ride. "What on earth is she doing?" I asked Tee Jay.

"Don't worry, Mum," he replied. "It looks like we have a lesbian budgerigar."

At this point I didn't know whether to laugh or cry, at Tee Jay's comments or the fact that the white female budgerigar was riding the female quails. I did neither and got up to make myself a cup of tea.

Today was June 3rd and it had been a while since I wrote anything down. I had been feeling very ill for several months and had suffered serious stomach cramps and pains that were quite scary. I would wake up night after night with pain and body sweats. Obviously because I was diabetic the sweats caused me to check my blood counts for sugar and they had always been OK. My doctor was convinced it was severe irritable bowel syndrome (IBS) and she was also convinced that writing my second book was causing me to have these problems due to the stress it brought. "Stop writing for a while, Bridget," she said, smiling at me. I replied, "But when it's flowing out, I might as well put it on paper as I am already thinking about it." I looked at her imploring her to agree with me. She sighed and leaning back in her chair nodded her head. "You do have a point, but you know what I mean." I smiled at her. She was a very pretty woman in her early thirties, and I often teased she should have been on the catwalk as she dressed immaculately too. Yet she was very articulate and clever, and I was pleased that she had chosen the profession she had. I stood up to go and after assuring her I would take care I left with a referral at my request for further investigations at the hospital.

The referral to the consultant, who I had seen years ago when he had first diagnosed the irritable bowel syndrome, was that he thought it was severe IBS and acid reflux, but he wasn't sure. He wanted me to have an endoscopy, which I refused as I knew I would be bolting out of the room and panicking. I explained my problem to him and he was very kind and understanding. His eyes twinkled as he told me that he could refer me for a barium meal instead. I hesitated and before I had said anything he told me that there would be only a couple of people in the room, and that it was nothing nasty and I should be out very quickly. I agreed and the date was set for the following week.

The day came and I already had problems: my diabetes was still unstable and Maggie had suggested I miss out on the evening base insulin so I would not go too low, as I couldn't eat until after the investigation. I was not booked in until 1pm and this was the earliest they could manage. As I set off with Joseph to the hospital I felt sick. "Oh, God," I said to him as he was driving. I had just taken a blood count for the sugar. "What is it?" He asked still concentrating on the road. He looked at me as we pulled up at the traffic lights. "It's only 4.5 and you know I can go under from 5," I said. I knew my blood sugar counter could be up to a whole unit out, and I always felt shaky and bad from under 5 and I was already just feeling a few of the signs. I was panicking. I had a sandwich with me but knew I couldn't eat. I shifted nervously in my seat, waiting for the sweating and palpitations. I knew I could battle on, and at times I had ignored the warnings until I had felt sleepy and shaky. I would then eat a biscuit or drink orange juice to get the sugar up quickly. I looked across at Joseph. "How long now?"

"We should be there in ten minutes." I clung on to my handbag and decided to hope for the best. We did arrive and booked ourselves in. The nurse came to take me pretty quickly and Joseph went to follow me through. She laughed . "Oh no, not you. We only want her lighting up at night." She winked at me as Joseph went to sit back down in the waiting room. After I had been given one of the awful hospital gowns where you are never sure which is the front or the back, I changed so I had the opening at my front, as I reckoned I would prefer to be aware if it became undone. I followed her through to the x-ray room. She started to ask me questions, but I knew that I had started to sweat and already had one palpitation. I interrupted her. "Sorry, but I am a diabetic and I have just started to go low." I didn't need to say any more: she had rushed out of the room to fetch the consultant in.

He came rushing in and took me over to this machine and asked me to stand on the step. I was given a massive spoonful of crystals to swallow and a drink. He said firmly, "Don't drink this until you have swallowed the crystals, as it might make you feel sick. You will want to belch, as it will produce gas when mixed." I looked distastefully at the massive heaped spoon of crystals that I was supposed to swallow. The drink was so small. I had not been allowed to drink all morning and my mouth was so dry. I placed the crystals in my mouth and tried my best to swallow. They stuck in my mouth and because I was so dry through nerves and not being able to drink, I struggled to swallow them. They reminded me of sherbet dabs, but instead of powder it was crystals. I swallowed and I swallowed, and he kept asking me if I had finished, and I smiled politely but all the time was trying to get this stuff down my throat without gagging. When I drank the fizzy drink, I had to turn my head away to attempt to belch discreetly and quietly, as he was right. It was like a fizz bomb exploding. If this wasn't enough I was then given a massive mug of what looked like thick mucus and told to drink it all. I started to drink it and hoped to down it in one go, but I had to stop twice. I was proud of myself that I kept it down. Then the whole stage I was on was tipped back so instead of standing I was lying on my back. The consultant was very caring he was asking me all the time if I was OK. I kept nodding. The next process was very undignified: I was asked to roll over onto my stomach and then to keep turning so I had done the full circle to end up back on my back. This was an attempt to make sure my stomach had been lined. I did as they asked, but it was like being in bed when you turn and your nightshirt gets caught. My gown kept getting stuck whilst at the same time I was trying to keep as dignified as I could and keep the gown closed. It was the nearest thing I had felt to being like a beached whale, and a breathless and sweaty one at that. I could laugh to myself because at the same time I was being photographed!

I managed to dress, and before we had even got out of the corridor I asked Joseph to bring me some water. I needed to drink. I rushed to the car and ate my sandwich. I felt sick but needed to get sugar into me as quickly as possible. The routine investigation had gone OK. I hadn't passed out or bolted, and I had stayed reasonably dignified. I was warned to drink as much water as I could for the next four days as otherwise my barium meal would impact and I would have a job to go to the toilet. I was also warned that when I went to the loo it would be white for a few days. It actually alarmed me, as for the next few days the residue I passed actually stuck in the loo, and it was very unpleasant getting rid of it. I drank loads of water, as I was thinking if that's what it did to the loo what was it doing to the insides of my body? I had hoped that the meds the consultant put me on would help, but the pain in my stomach was terrible and even worse was the burning sensation in my throat. It also made me breathless. I am ashamed I felt quite sorry for myself, as I was still adjusting to being a diabetic and missed my sugar. Now as I was told I had acid reflux I was warned not to eat a lot of other foods or drinks. Tea and coffee were a no-go, and fizzy drinks were out, along with citrus drinks and dairy food. I ended up on water and virtually brown bread and rice. I was feeling miserable and also worried as we were due to fly out to Portugal. I had opted to go private as I was in such pain, and as I returned to the consultant, I asked him if I could have my money back as the meds hadn't worked. I laughed, as I was joking. He looked at me and with those same twinkling eyes said, "You just sound like my wife." We both laughed. He doubled my meds and booked me in for a scan. I was due to have the scan the day before we went on holiday.

We were on the plane to Portugal. My scan had been fine, and I had been told it was severe acid reflux combined with IBS and given some more meds. I was relieved and glad that I had an answer. The plane roared and the wings shook as we started to pick up speed on the runway. I was scared. I didn't like flying, as I felt powerless and I always had the thought 'What if' in the back of my mind. The plane was rattling and Jo Jo turned round and said, "Did you pick the cheapest flight you could find?" It was a statement more than a question, but it so made me laugh as the answer was yes, and in those seconds as we lifted off and the engines were roaring, and the plane rattling, I questioned the wisdom of my choice. As I laughed Jo Jo did as well, and I thought I have to remember that one. I turned to look behind us. Tee Jay was staring out of the window and Joseph was leaning back with his eyes shut.

The signs flashed and it was OK to lower the tables in front of the seats, and I immediately reached for my book. We had been to Portugal for the last five years and stayed in the same villa. The owners were lovely people called Tess and Tony and we felt lucky to have found the place. We had our own private pool, a big resort next door where we could use the facilities such as the tennis courts, and the beach was five minutes by car. We were also lucky as the people at the restaurant next door had been very friendly. The lighthouse was just down the road and we went for walks down there. The beach nearby was a typical one for the area: it was reached by going down many steps and then walking through caves to the secluded bay. We preferred this one to going into Carvoeiro. We went into Carvoeiro in the daytime, or in the evening to visit the small shops and to have a drink looking out to the sea.

This year I had just built a Facebook page for my book and had my new Kindle to hand, and was able to read the many messages. I was astonished to read that someone had nominated my book for the Open University book of the month for July and August. It was a big privilege and I felt very humbled. I also received some supportive messages from a man called Patrick who had appreciated the site and my book. He was later to become a good friend. It was a nice feeling to know that my book had created such a positive influence for people. We celebrated both Tee Jay's and Joseph's birthdays, and had a lot of fun especially as all the people at the restaurant joined in singing *Happy Birthday* on both occasions. Joseph always teased Tee Jay, who didn't like seafood, by pointing his shrimps with eyes on his plate facing him. He also teased him about the local *frango piri piri*, as our poultry-loving Tee Jay wouldn't eat chicken. The next day we travelled down the road to the local beach and climbed down the hundred steps through the caves to the sand and sea. The sun was bright and a little breeze rippled through the sun parasols. I lazily watched the kids play beach ball until we all decided to take the plunge. Somehow we had made a pact that none of us would back out of going into the sea once we started to go in. The coldness of the water made me gasp, but I continued to wade in until I was swimming out behind Jo Jo.

Later we were all sunbathing on the beach mats when I suddenly realised I had forgotten to bring a snack with me. I cursed silently to myself and wondered if my sugar levels would stay OK. I thought about the numerous steps up to the top of the cliff and closed my eyes, really angry with myself. As the time got on to one o'clock, I started to feel the warning signs that my body needed sugar. My heart was having palpitations and I was sweating even more, which was not due to the sun. I reluctantly turned to Joseph. "We shall have to go." He immediately stood up, rolling the towels up into the bag. The kids followed, shaking their beach mats, and Tee Jay grabbed the parasol as Jo Jo held on to the beach mats. We trundled across the sand to the cave entrance, each of us grimacing as the heat of the sun radiated through the white sand to the soles of our feet.

By the time I reached the top of the cliff my legs were shaky and I felt out of breath. It was a hard climb anyway, and I knew it was ludicrous to have attempted it with a hypo coming on. I grinned at the kids and hoped that my dilemma was hidden. As soon as we reached the villa I headed inside for some of my glucose tablets and sank onto the chair in the shade, relieved I had made it back

Once home I wanted to say hello to Asti and Amba. They both wouldn't stop crying and whining in excitement and I got down on my knees to hug them both. They responded by lying on their backs, tail wagging and then jumping up and down and running around in circles, barking like mad. I had already seen some of the cats, and Tee Jay went out to check on his hens. Only after we knew everyone was OK did we settle for a drink and to start unpacking. I received a shock when I saw Bella, as she was so huge, and heart in mouth I realised she was pregnant.

The days passed quickly and the children didn't see much of the sun. The rest of the holidays were cloudy, dull with the odd rainy day. I tried to spend some time with Jo Jo and Tee Jay, yet I was also busy revising for my psychology degree. My final exam after seven years of hard work with the Open University was in October and I knew I needed to achieve a merit for a 1.1 first-class honours psychology degree. Dr Lynn asked me why a 1.1 meant so much. He explained to me that most people would be happy just to gain a degree.

***

"Why, Bridget?"

I looked across at him and shrugged my shoulders. I had always been competitive, and this was no different. "Well, firstly when someone tells you not to expect to gain a first because only clever people achieve that, and only people like her son who went to a private school gain firsts, well, that got under my skin even though she said that she meant it well, as I wasn't happy with my marks at the time and she was trying to be kind." I stuck my chin out defiantly. "Secondly, my sister told me that I wouldn't be accepted into university because I hadn't got any A-levels, and just because I wanted to prove to myself what I could achieve if I tried my hardest."

Dr Lynn sat back and smiled. I looked at him defiantly. I could see no wrong in wanting to try my hardest, and whatever the outcome I would always know I had given it my best shot. He then said with a laugh, "And what if you fail?"

I laughed because as he was laughing, and I didn't reply. I knew I had mixed feelings about my psychology degree, for if I gained a first, I knew I would be very happy. Yet I also knew I would be thinking what I could have done if I had managed to have the chance of studying all those years back. Then my senses kicked in, for I loved the kids and Joseph, and to me I wouldn't change any of this for the world so my past was package and parcel of where I was today. When I first started to study, my first course was on health and social care, and I wasn't sure whether to follow this direction. Yet I turned to psychology, as I was curious to learn more about the mind and why people behaved the way they did. I enjoyed learning throughout the degree and smiled as Dr Lynn joked that I should have done a course on something else like gardening.

***

As Sam had worked hard throughout the spring to get used to our animals so that she and Tom could look after them when we went to Portugal, I managed to learn a lot more about her, and also she and Tom became much

69

closer friends to us than before. Tom made me laugh, as he was a tough young man with a cheeky grin. Although he would stand up to a lad twice his age, our cockerel John soon had him running and jumping over the fence to escape being attacked. John was a white cockerel who we had hatched in an incubator. The older he got the more he ruled the roost, and in the spring time he became very aggressive to any intruder who approached his hens, including us. It was no joke when he first attacked Tee Jay, as he drew blood and pecked some gashing holes to the bone where Tee Jay was left screaming in pain. It was the first time I had doubts about whether I wanted to keep one of our animals, yet it was Tee Jay who pleaded and begged Joseph and I to let him keep John. Over time John became more docile, but was still aggressive at times. Sam and Tom helped us build some pens and dig a pond out before we went to Portugal, and it was during this time that Sam became a good friend of Pumpkin, our Sebastopol Frizzle goose.

The geese had been a newish venture of mine, and although I had originally ordered a trio, unfortunately we had ended up with three males. It had taken nearly two years to sort them out, as geese are very hard to sex. In the end we ended up with Goldie and Leah, who became a pair, and another female called Beattie, who should have paired up with Pumpkin. Unfortunately Pumpkin from a very young age had decided he preferred human company to his fellow geese. Beattie ended up with Goldie and Leah, and Pumpkin preferred to stroll about on his own and creep up to any of us who ventured into the paddock. Unfortunately it didn't end there: he would creep up to the back of you and if you bent down for anything he would not miss a chance to become more friendly. I still laugh now, as it was comical. Sam was helping me saw a piece of wood and as she bent down to hold the wood Pumpkin took his chance. I hadn't been looking, but all I heard was Sam squeal loudly and jump up quickly. "I haven't had an offer like that for years," she joked to me, rubbing her bottom. Pumpkin had pecked her hard and she had brushed him off, but she found it hilarious and we both rolled about on the ground laughing as Pumpkin looked on, pleased with himself. There was many a time I was hammering or working on an aviary and my friendly goose would stand beside me. I always had to remember to face him as I bent down to pick up some tools. I would also say, "No" quite loudly and he would seriously hesitate and wander a few paces back.

Pumpkin became very popular with our friends, and Sam even thought of having a Sebastopol goose at her house. She had to reluctantly agree that it would not be suitable, as they were very loud, and she lived on an estate where someone would be bound to complain about the noise.

Besides making a pond for the ducks, we also made a new cage for the chipmunks. I called it the Tardis, as it was shaped like one. We decided it would look good opposite the lounge patio doors, where we could see it when we were sitting down. Also it was beside the bird aviary and in the area where we sat to enjoy a drink in the evening. I still had my old male Roland

and decided to get two whites and two more striped females. I had been keeping chipmunks for the last thirty years and had even freelanced in magazines about their care. Sam liked them and reckoned that once she got sorted out she would like to keep them as well.

It was August 22nd 2011, and the day after what would have been my dad's birthday. Tee Jay turned to me. "Mum, I forgot to say Bella wanted to come out of the shower room so I let her out." I looked up quickly. "Crumbs, Tee, are you sure she is alright? She is due to have her kittens anytime, and I thought that's why we were keeping her to her bed in there."

Tee Jay looked at me. "Mum, she asked. She was scratching at the door." He looked at me, waiting for a response. "OK, but just for a short while as we have our dinner, then you can put her back." As if on cue Bella strolled into the lounge, and lay on the carpet and started to wash herself. I went back into the kitchen and started to dish out the dinner. "Jo Jo, please set the table. Tee, can you help carry, please?" Both kids appeared, and as Jo Jo set the table in the lounge Tee helped me carry the dishes through. It was lasagne and chips, and I had just started to eat my chips when Tee shouted out, "Mum, Bella has a mouse. She has gone behind the chair." I grabbed a chip and darted for the chair and looked over the top to see if I could rescue the poor little mouse. "Oh no," I gasped. "What?" both kids chorused. I was too busy trying to balance the cushions behind the chair. Tee climbed up and also gasped. This made Jo Jo abandon her plate and the three of us stared in disbelief. Bella was panting, extending and pushing hard. Tee's mouse turned out to be a newly born kitten still wet from birth, balanced precariously on the pile of cushions behind the chair. As we all watched another popped out and Bella immediately started to lick it. She started to strain again and I jumped into action, not having time to panic. "Tee, run and get a cardboard box. Jo Jo run and get some newspapers." Both kids shot off and I surveyed the scene. It wasn't good, as already one of the newborns rolled down the back of the pile of cushions and Bella stood up with another appearing. *Shit, shit, shit!* I didn't say it, but I was thinking it. I knew that I shouldn't handle them, as she might reject them, but there was hardly any choice as another appeared. I had to pull the chair out with the risk of some falling off the cushion, but I had to get there to rescue the one from the back. "Quick, pull the chair slowly towards you. Do not push it, just pull." I surprised myself as I spoke calmly to Tee although I felt like screaming inside. Tee was good and as he pulled the chair I propped up the cushion with Bella and the two kittens. Jo Jo placed the cardboard box with flattened newspapers next to me. "Good girl." I carefully and quickly picked up one of the kittens and placed it into the box. I hoped Bella would follow, bringing the other, but she didn't. She ran to the box, jumped in, and carried the kitten back out to the cushion. "Shit." Ashamedly I swore out loud in front of my kids, but I was now worried for the one at the back. "Quick, Tee, as I put both these in the box pick up Bella carefully and place her in gently but

71

quickly too." I grabbed both kittens, but before Tee could move Bella followed and jumped in as well. I ignored her, lifted the cushion and rescued the one at the back. It was huddled onto a cushion below; I quickly placed it in the box just as Bella went to jump out again with another. She hesitated and luckily decided with three kittens in the box she could settle in there. I breathed a deep sigh of relief as Jo Jo went, "Yuck, look at that!"

Bella was giving birth again and it wasn't a pretty sight: the sac was thick and this kitten looked like a messy blob and headless. I nearly heaved, but when Bella started to lick and remove the outer, it turned out fine. It was a little tortoiseshell to go along with a couple of gingers and a black and white kitten. Our dinners remained cold. I couldn't face eating lasagne and chips, and especially ketchup, after facing this, and both the kids felt the same. "Go on, Tee, go and clear the ketchup up," Jo Jo was teasing him. Tee pulled a face as he took the plates back into the kitchen. Amba and Asti looked on with eager eyes. He fed the dogs and returned. "How many, Mum?"

"Five so far," I replied. "Another dark one, and it looks like there is another on the way. "I think she will have six." Both kids smiled. I had told them to sit down and leave Bella in peace. I had placed the box behind the chair so she felt secure and both Tee Jay and Jo Jo turned to watch the television.

It was just past ten, both kids had gone to bed and Bella had done me proud: seven kittens – another tortoiseshell and another ginger. So she had three gingers, two darkish and two tortoiseshells. I stayed up to let Joseph know and he was delighted when he came in. "How's my girl?" he whispered as he looked into the box. Bella was too busy licking and washing them. The newspaper was dirty, but I didn't want to disturb her. "I'll change it tomorrow. Keep the dogs out of here." We went to bed excited about the new additions to our household. The next morning I got up early and crept downstairs. I hoped that all the kittens had survived as the last was tiny. I was amazed, as when I counted Bella had produced another ginger. so we had four gingers and eight kittens in all.

"You clever girl," I whispered to my cat, and I stroked her head. I was so proud of her. I felt guilty too, as we had booked her in to be neutered but she had caught us out and she was still so young to be a mum. I brought her some food in and fresh water and went to make myself a cup of tea. It was a few hours later when the children got up and both were happy when they saw the new addition. I went and made a big fuss of Amba and Asti, as I didn't want the dogs to feel left out. I then turned my attention to our other cats.

The summer holidays passed so quickly and it was frustrating when the kids went back to school as we had kept waiting for the summer to arrive and it was as if it never did. The weather had been chilly, rainy and quite gloomy. It affected our moods and we were all a bit fed up. Bella and the kittens continued to thrive and I took great delight in posting the photos up on my Facebook page.

I settled down to revise for my psychology degree, and I was panicking as I realised after seven years that I could still fail my target for a first-class honours at my last hurdle. A merit was a mark above 70 in the tutor-marked assignments, and I also had to get a 70 or more in the exam. It was also much harder as my memory wasn't so good. I did what I usually did, and wrote pages and pages. I also bought revision cards, and I used them. I used different coloured pens and I went over and over, pulling out different pieces, and the more I took the time to concentrate the more it sank in and made sense.

I was lucky as the Open University had supported me all the way. I was allowed a home exam as I would not have coped or been able to attend an official place. I already had a job to cope with a stranger coming into my house, let alone being restricted to three hours in the same room, and I requested a female invigilator and also asked if it was possible for me to be introduced to her first. The Open University took all my needs on board and I was very fortunate to have the same invigilator for all my exams. The very first time she came out she scared me and asked to synchronise watches. Already in my head I had a nickname for her: 'The Sergeant Major'. She was very kind but also very professional, and I still had to show my passport for identity to her in the following years. She sat on the sofa with her paperwork whilst I sat at a table next to her in my lounge. I was allowed rest breaks and half an hour extra time. I needed them as I still suffered from ME and obviously when stressed, which was high at exam time, I still suffered flashbacks and had to fight to keep grounded from my post-traumatic stress disorder. It made me think back to when I suffered an unexpected setback.

***

Flashback:
I walked into the hospital to see Dr Lynn. I felt restless and desperate, but I didn't know why. As I sat near him beside the desk, I was uneasy and he sensed there was something wrong. I couldn't speak, but the intensity was so deep it was firing through me. I felt so bad I wanted to sit on the floor. I felt that it would not be enough. I would need to go through it. I couldn't stay still: I needed to go, I needed to escape, but I had no idea how to escape from how I was feeling. I reached out and grabbed the cuff of his suit.

"I'll ring for Andrea. Do you want Andrea down here?" He was already dialling the number and there was a sense of urgency in the room. There was a knock at the door and Andrea walked in. She pulled up a chair and smiled at me. She asked me what I had been doing at the weekend. I started to tell her about walking around the lakes behind our house with Tee Jay and Jo Jo.

"It was supposed to be a nice walk. I had both the dogs, and the children were playing as we walked around." The words were spilling out fast and garbled. Andrea was nodding as she listened to me. Dr Lynn sat to my side and Andrea was nearly opposite me. I continued. "There were a few fishermen about and I had to watch Amba, as she was always running over to them to get their sandwiches. Asti had to be kept on a lead as she was over-protective when we went out. It was warm and…"

I stopped and fell back in my chair. I stared at Andrea. "What are you doing here? Why are you here?" I stared hard at her. Andrea suddenly looked panicked. Dr Lynn interrupted.

"What do you mean, Bridget? You know I asked Andrea to come. You saw me pick up the phone, and you agreed to her coming, remember?" He was looking intently at me, and Andrea looked so scared,. She spoke to me. "You look awful. What's happening?" As she spoke, Dr Lynn had already come over to me. "I am just going to take your pulse, Bridget." As he held my wrist, I was aware that I had slumped back in my chair and that I could not feel my head. It was as if it was made of cardboard. I was vaguely aware that I was trying to feel it with my hand but had no sensation and it was like all the pressure was just seeping out of my body and taking my life with it. I couldn't move and could hear them telling each other to move me over to a big chair. Between them both they managed to transfer me across the room from the small chair I was on to a bigger chair. I fell where I was placed, aware they were in the room but completely out of it. Andrea was asking if I wanted a cup of sweet tea, and Dr Lynn agreed for her to go and make one. I sat and stared like a cabbage, with eyes not moving but aware of what was happening. Dr Lynn was saying, "I'll go and get someone off the ward and make sure there's a bed free."

As they both left the room, I knew unless I struggled to get up and out I would be detained. I wanted to get back home, yet I didn't want that awful feeling again, and I was scared. I managed somehow to stand up and move myself over to the door. As I turned the handle it already pushed towards me and Tim entered the room. I liked Tim. He was one of my favourite nurses off the ward. "Hey, where are you off to? Come and sit down." By now my legs had turned to jelly and I nearly fell back into the larger chair. Andrea walked in with a cup of tea for me and Dr Lynn appeared behind her. I felt very woozy and my head felt full of cotton wool. They gave me a few minutes to drink my tea and then started to escort me to the ward. As I entered the corridor I was like a sheep being herded into a pen. They were making for the ward and I tried to make for the exit to the stairs. "Don't be silly, Bridget," Dr Lynn said, and Andrea nodded, raising her eyebrows at me. Tim linked his arm in mine and actually I needed the support as I could hardly walk. I allowed myself to be led onto the ward and was trying to clear my head to think how Joseph would react. I already knew he would not be pleased. I tried to argue verbally and refused to allow myself to be admitted. They told me off for being silly, but I wanted to go home to be back with the kids. I ended up being sectioned and was in hospital yet again.

Marked dissociation.

I was on level ones and I had a nurse at an arm's length twenty-four hours a day. The nurse as usual changed every hour and the first nurse I had was Shirley. She was nice and I had guessed her age to be early sixties. She made me a cup of tea and I'd needed one. I still felt very odd, and couldn't feel my head. Dr Lynn had called my episode a 'marked dissociation'. I guessed it meant that I had dissociated and it was called 'marked' as it had been witnessed. I might not have got it right, but that was my interpretation of it. I wasn't happy I was back in hospital, and Joseph even less so. Yet Dr Lynn was worried that it might happen again, and as I clearly had no control of it, I could understand why I was not allowed home. Although I didn't want to be there, inside of me part of me was relieved, as I knew I had felt such an intense despair that I couldn't control it. I didn't feel depressed as such. I didn't want to die; I didn't want to curl in a corner and hide. I wanted to get home to see Jo Jo and Tee Jay, yet I knew when I was at home I couldn't cope. I did have a feeling that I wanted to sink to the ground, and yet even that wasn't low enough. I had felt so desperate I had grabbed Dr Lynn's sleeve, yet I didn't know how to stop it or handle it. I had been scared, as I was doing my best to hold it together, but the intensity of the feelings was so strong it took over. I didn't want to go and jump over a cliff to end it all. I was fighting with all my strength for it to go away. I didn't know what difference the hospital would make, and part of me felt safer, as it was like I had some sort of safety net. But I also knew that the restraint would place pressure on me in certain ways and that at times I would do anything to get away because my freedom was curtailed. My state was unpredictable and I would act out impulsively.

I took any chance or opportunity that came my way without thinking it through. I was on high alert in the hospital, every sense tuned in to react to the slightest stimulation. I would look eagerly at the timetable of the nurses' rota, and without intentionally planning it I would automatically take in who was doing what and where they would be. Any significant factors would be taken into account, such as when the trolley man came with the newspapers and which patients would most likely be in the reception area. Any slightest detail that would give me an opportunity to increase my self-protection as I saw it, I noted. My self-protection included taking any piece of cutlery that was available, and these would be snapped at the slightest opportunity, or if I got bored. It would serve as a challenge when I had a nurse at arm's length to be able to hide and snap the cutlery whilst they were there. It was possible, as most nurses at some point would chat to another patient or nurse, or turn their attention away from me to read a magazine or watch the television in my room. As long as I was sitting quietly they took it for granted that I was behaving. I felt guilty at times, as part of me knew it was wrong, but again to me it was a necessity. I used the knives to undo any screw I could find. I stored and smashed any mug or plate I could get hold of. 'Sharps' as they were called in the hospital were items that could be used to cut with. When I was first admitted I was asked if I had any sharps and I honestly didn't know what they were. This was even when I had entered, hiding five razor blades in my mobile phone casing. These hadn't been found, but later I had told Dr Lynn where they were. Besides the cutlery and mugs, I took anything that could be adapted to be a sharp: this could be a drawing pin, a paperclip, a little piece of wire. Anything plastic could be used. I was that desperate even on walks around the hospital that I would pick up broken glass and store it. It was strange, as before I had been admitted to hospital I would not have dreamed of picking up a piece of glass or smashing a mug. This was a completely different environment, and I adapted by using anything that made me feel secure. I also tried to self-strangle by tying anything that would do around my neck and tightening it as hard as I could. I had a few narrow escapes, including one where I did lose consciousness. I was not behaving rationally but could not see it at the time.

"Come on, Bridget, let's play scrabble with Kim," said Tracey, who was the nurse on duty now. I had been asked earlier if I would play and I had reluctantly agreed to the challenge even though I hated the game. It was at least something to do. I followed Tracey to the lounge. I first looked to make sure there was hardly anybody in and chose the table near the door. Tracey laughed. "Don't think I haven't noticed. I am watching you like a hawk!" I looked up to her grinning face; her eyes were bright and her freckles matched her red hair. I shuffled my chair and she half rose. I pulled it into the table and started to arrange the board. Kim had joined us; she had been admitted again for manic depression. She was usually singing and dancing around and teasing all the nurses, or chatting all the young doctors up when they entered the ward. She started to arrange the tiles and she made me laugh as she made some very colourful words up. "Excuse my French," she said, laughing in her chair. I realised that this was not going to be a serious game and looked across to Tracey who was shaking her head but also laughing.

It was about an hour or so later that I realised I didn't feel too well. I looked across to Melanie as Tracey my nurse had finished her hour, and it was now Melanie who was looking after me. I stared at her hard, my mind blank. I just stared at Melanie again. "Are you OK, Bridget?" she asked.

I nodded and stared at her. I didn't want to admit it, but she suddenly looked far away. It was a strange feeling and I reached out to feel the table, as everything seemed unreal. It seemed strange, as although I wanted to reach out, my arm wouldn't move naturally and I had to really concentrate to make my arm move. It was like looking at my arm and at the thing on the end of it, which was my hand, but I didn't feel it belonged to me. I watched this hand touch the table and I could suddenly see myself sitting at the table.

Melanie had got up and she was coming over to this dark-haired girl. She touched and guided me gently on the arm. "Come on, let's go back to your room." I watched her guide me back to my room. She sat me on the bed and shouted down the corridor for another nurse. I realised that I had that funny feeling back where my head felt like cardboard, and I was trying to move my arm with the thing on the end of it to feel if my head was still on my shoulders. I had made contact but with minimal feeling, and the loss of sensation was frightening. I tried to pull myself back against the pillow. It is strange to describe, but I felt detached and unreal. I wasn't looking down at myself anymore; I was staring at Melanie. She called out to Tracey, "Can you make Bridget a cup of tea, two sugars, and make me a coffee? And be as quick as you can, thanks." She shut the door and came and sat on a chair next to my bed. I still stared at her and I just felt that I was staring through my eyes and that the rest of my body did not exist. I had to concentrate hard to get my hand on one of my arms to pinch the other arm. I could see myself doing it but I could not feel the result.

It was a couple of minutes later when Tracey walked in with my tea and Melanie's coffee. Melanie thanked her and put my tea onto the little chest of drawers next to my bed. I did not dare hold it, as I still could not feel anything throughout my body. Melanie was very calm. She had not asked or spoken to me but had let me relax on the bed. I gradually decided to have a go at drinking my tea; Melanie put her coffee down and held the cup with me. If she had not I would have dropped it. I sipped at the hot liquid slowly, thankful that I could taste it, and very slowly I started to feel my body again.

Melanie waited until I had finished my tea, and then brushing back her dark brown hair, she asked, "What was going on, Bridge?"

I shrugged my shoulders and shook my head. "All I know is that all of a sudden you were in the distance and getting further away. I lost all sense of feelings and it was as if I was in the distance watching both of us from somewhere else." I realised as I spoke that my voice had got quieter and that as I said it, I realised how daft it sounded, but I could only describe how it felt.

Melanie picked up her mug and mine and told me to rest. "I'll see you in the morning. I am on first shift." She smiled at me. I smiled back and watched as she beckoned another nurse to come into my room before she left.

I tossed and turned in my bed. Tonight the nurse had chosen to sit by the bed, and other times nurses would sit at the door. Who would sit where was a lottery system, as it depended on who was in charge and on the nurse. This inconsistency could have an effect on how you felt: sometimes I wanted the nurse to be as near as possible as it made me feel safer. Other times, I wanted to scream at them to go away.

I missed Jo Jo and Tee Jay, and Joseph would ring every day at 4pm and put both the children on the phone. Tee Jay would hardly say anything, but I could sense he clung on to every word I said. "You be a good boy. It won't be long before I am home. I think you have to show Daddy Lioney." I tried my hardest to keep my voice cheerful, and it was harder with Tee Jay as I had to keep talking. Lioney was his favourite toy, a soft cuddly lion. Jo Jo was easier as she chatted away and it gave me time to pull myself together. It wasn't easy being away from my children, and although I enjoyed the telephone contact, it tore me to pieces. Joseph was so busy he didn't have time to get too emotional, as he had a business to run and two children to look after, including all the animals, and he also tried to visit me whenever he could. We had decided that it was impractical for the children to visit me in the week and they only came at weekends. This was for two main reasons: one was the time commitment as Joseph was so busy, and the other was that I thought it would be too upsetting for the children and myself to keep meeting in the week, as it was fantastic when we first saw each other, but when the time came to say goodbye, both children would get upset and it was so hard for me.

Today I had walked to the restaurant with my nurse. It wasn't because I was hungry, but more of a chance to get away from the ward and to have a change of scenery. Whilst we queued up at the till to pay for our drinks, Tina my nurse walked in front of me and paid. I didn't protest anymore, as the staff got a discount and some of the nurses would insist on paying, and then I paid them back. I was sitting chatting to her and drinking my hot chocolate, watching the news when suddenly I felt a bit strange. She started to look further away than she was. I had read that high-anxiety episodes could give you a similar feeling, yet I had been laughing and chatting. I turned round to her. "When we have finished the drinks, can we walk around the long way back to the ward?"

"Yes, yes course we can, but no running off."

I shook my head. It was the last thing on my mind. Five minutes later we were walking around the maternity unit watching the grey squirrels darting through the trees. I thought some fresh air and a walk would do me good, but I was wrong: halfway round I felt so weak and ill. Tina and I had been chatting, but now I hadn't the energy and I needed it to get back. Tina realised, as I also was very hesitant in speaking. The truth was I went to speak but the words would not come out. I spoke in half sentences without finishing them and Tina looked at me. "Come on, let's get you back to the ward." She placed her hand on my elbow as if for support. I now had to concentrate on my walking, on making each foot move after the other. I didn't like what was happening and the more I panicked the worse it got. Once on the ward, I didn't look at anyone. I headed straight for my room and lay down on my bed. Tina followed me and I could tell she was worried, yet I hadn't got the strength to be bothered. I lay flat out and hadn't even taken my coat off. Tina called out to one of the nurses passing. "Can you bring the blood pressure monitor?" She turned and shouted after them, "And stick the kettle on. We will have two teas here."

My blood pressure was fine, and after resting I started to feel a bit better. I didn't like what was happening, as felt I had no control over it. I just hoped that it would pass in time.

***

I looked at all the questions for the exam and soon realised that I could answer most of them, and I wasted time deciding which ones to go for. I used my dad's Parker, which was a pledge I had made to myself before I started my degree. My dad had died in 1999, and it had been very tough. I had helped my mum nurse him daily for his final six months. Tee Jay was only nine months old and Jo Jo two-and-a-half. We had managed, but it was heart rending: I loved my dad so much, and when we found out the awful news that he had pancreatic cancer, I had made a decision that I wanted to spend every second possible with him. I didn't have many of dad's possessions when he died, but mum had given me his pen and I cherished it. It had made sense to use it for my degree and I think he would have liked that. Each time I had started my exam I had whispered a silent message to him and today was no different. "Wish me luck, Dad," I whispered, and I grasped his pen and started to write.

I was positioned so that I could look out of my patio doors in the lounge towards the paddock, and as I sat writing, there was a commotion from the paddocks and I could see Pumpkin trying to fight with Goldie through the fencing. I looked at the Sergeant Major. She hadn't noticed, and I told myself off and settled down to the exam. I had three one-hour essays to write and I was fortunate that I was allowed rest breaks in between due to my disabilities. I had divided these breaks up and once I had finished the first question would ask politely if I could have a break. The Sergeant Major was so professional, logging the time in her book, and would then stand up and follow me into the kitchen. This close monitoring made me think of the hospital, and I was very relieved she didn't insist on coming into the bathroom when I went to the toilet, although she did do a thorough inspection beforehand of the bathroom to make sure I couldn't cheat. Cheating really wasn't my sort of thing, as even with kids' games I wouldn't cheat, as if and when I won I wanted to know I had done it on my own merit, and to me if I cheated I would never have known if I could have achieved it without cheating. I disliked cheats, as I always thought that they cheated themselves more than anyone else.

I felt quite emotional finishing my exam. Not only was I saying goodbye to the Open University, which had been a magnificent experience, I was also saying goodbye to my Sergeant Major whose professionalism I had had the privilege of experiencing for each and every one of my exams. She had also bought my book and I had a lot of respect for her as she had been kind yet strict. I was delighted when through mutual agreement we decided to keep in touch.

It felt surreal when the exam was over. After seven years of studying, I was suddenly free. I didn't know what to do with myself. I started to pick up all the revision scraps of paper that were around the house to throw them away in the bin. I phoned my mum up to let her know I had finished. "I did my best, Mum. I couldn't have done any more. I know I have passed but don't know if I have done enough for a merit. It's no use worrying: what will be, will be."

"Well done, love," my mum said, and I knew she was proud of me whatever the outcome. Besides Mum being proud, I was surprised at the number of kind messages I received from people on my Facebook site.

CHAPTER TEN – FACEBOOK SITE

My Facebook page for the book never ceased to amaze me. It was originally created to promote my book, and then grew socially. I made many new friends on the page, and also received numerous messages about child abuse. The accounts shocked me, as I never realised how widespread child abuse was. As an increasing number of people joined, so did the messages. Some of these messages brought home how mental health issues were not being dealt with in the UK, and how many of these people were like silent heroes battling through on their own. These accounts sadly did not surprise me, as I had been informed that mental health care was way down the list relating to other areas in the medical world and that resources were tight. I understood why the Victorian stigma about mental health was still around. It was ironic, as technology and other areas had moved forward with the times, yet still the people with the power and resources to bring mental health issues up to date still hid behind this stigma. It angered and frustrated me, as on the one hand mental health issues were increasing, and on the other no one was doing anything about it. I wondered if someday somebody among the powers that be might just realise that if mental health was supported more, through successful management and understanding some of the issues could be tackled and eventually it would not only be the decent thing to do but it would be cost-effective. Child abuse was just one significant issue, and I personally was horrified that more people in the appropriate areas were not taking enough action to promote awareness and to help stop this terrible action. The main issues that stood out from these messages were because of the stigma about mental health many of the sufferers not only had to battle through on their own, they had to fight against people who should have known better but through lack of education did not, and gave wrong management and wrong support. Even loved ones close to the sufferer closed their eyes and pretended it wasn't happening, and those who tried to help often could not give enough support as they didn't understand enough and did not have the correct backing. The consequences of all of this are that people who were suffering felt alone, became more depressed and their illnesses lingered. Other symptoms and long-term effects were low self-esteem and feeling guilty. Frustration doesn't even to start to cover it when it is clear that with the correct support a lot of these issues could be avoided. The discrimination – and that was the word that fitted into my head – was widespread. Examples of this are that people with physical disabilities are praised and thrown into the limelight because their personal battles against their disability could be seen. How many times do you see a person with a mental health disability even probably sometimes fighting to stay alive being praised or made an example of? It actually angered me, as when I received messages from so many people who have had to fight so hard on their own without support then these people should be recognised. It is no wonder they have low self-esteem and hide away. I am thankful that people with physical disabilities are praised and their strength and battles recognised. Some of the soldiers who come back with limbs lost deserve the recognition and appreciation, but so do many others who have mental impairments who have to battle on silently. I actually feel sickened when I think about it. I applaud anyone with a disability who is trying to overcome it, and so respect the people who are trying to fight for more awareness for mental health issues and wish more could be done.

Whilst I write about the messages I received, many of which were shocking, sad and in some cases tragic as with support they could have been avoided, I noticed that there was a huge problem with awareness for men who had been abused. Again it was down to stigma: men are supposed to be strong and powerful and the image of a male being abused has different consequences than for a female. Yet this should not take away the significance, and it was hard for a man to admit that he had been abused and to also externalise this distress. I had many messages of praise for the insight my book gave to child abuse, and I hope that more men will be able to write about their accounts to provide vital insight and hopefully more men can come forward and receive the support they are entitled to.

My Facebook site is still growing, and has also taught me a lot about people. The reviews I received for my book on Amazon had mostly been positive, yet obviously some people disliked the book – some probably had issues themselves and projected their frustrations and issues in the reviews. It was sad to read how close-minded some people were. The book was criticised for the grammar, as I had been let down, but for people to advise others not to buy the book as they didn't like it went beyond me when the medics had praised it to be of help, and so many people had sent messages of thanks after it helped turn their life around. I suppose it depended what was weighted as important.

Confidence was one of the main issues in all of the messages I received – this and feeling isolated and alone. Both of these could be understood due to the management of mental health, and the old-fashioned stigma that still hung around today. The Facebook site introduced me to new friends, and I soon gathered that the community that belonged to my site was not only people who had suffered abuse. There were many professionals such as counsellors, psychologists and therapists. Alongside these were psychology students and many other people who had an interest in mental health. This demonstrated hope that people did want to gain insight, learn more and to even voice their opinions about mental health. I was careful to make sure the site wasn't overloaded with mental health issues and problems. I introduced the occasional blog, promoted the book and posted entertaining messages containing photographs, positivity and beauty. The site received many private messages from people who had suffered from abuse. It also received some encouragement and compliments from people studying mental health. The significance of the site was that most of the feedback and communication was about caring, whether it be towards humans or animals. It sent out a positive message that people do care, could be warm-hearted and were capable of being loving.

Sadly it was demonstrated on my site through the messages I received from many people, that because of abuse that had happened in their earlier years they had suffered from mental health problems and yet hadn't received the correct support. Many people reported that their families knew the abuse was happening but still chose to look the other way. It was understandable in some cases, as the abuser was the strongest member of the household, while in other cases it was kept quiet because of the shame. In some tragic cases it was because the whole family were involved. It amazed me how the person had survived and continued with their life. It made me angry because through the nature of child abuse the suppressed feelings had consequences down the line, and although these survivors were trying their hardest, they still lacked support from the appropriate authorities and the stigma about mental health meant that resources were low and in some areas non-existent. The other issue was that even loved ones and friends didn't support as well as they could, because of the lack of awareness and education on mental health. Many people still do not know how to support, manage or react to mental health issues. People are more worried about the embarrassment and what others will think than about the survivor's welfare. This is never going to change when the people who could do something about it will not. It will only change when someone close to someone in authority suffers a similar experience and then change may happen, or the person in authority will do the same as everyone else go into denial and pretend it didn't happen. As I write this I know some of it is repeated, but to catch awareness, sometimes one has to push hard!

Soon after I had written my book, I sent it to the Chief Executive of the Local NHS Partnership Trust. I hadn't really expected a response, yet I received a letter inviting me to talk about the book, and it gave me a chance to draw upon some care issues I had received whilst I was in the psychiatric unit.

***

CHAPTER ELEVEN – THE ROUND TABLE

I drove into the car park glancing to my right. The brick building looked formidable in the sunlight and the big bay windows at the front enhanced the air of esteem that seemed to surround the place. I guessed the history behind the buildings and the fact that it was the local NHS Partnership Trust headquarters gave it this official status. I drove up the track, easily parked my car and sat back.

I had arrived early and was not too hasty to enter the building. I lazed back in my seat and looked around; several people were arriving. I guessed some to be staff returning after lunch, and others looked like first-time arrivals, as they walked this way and that scanning the place for directions.

I took a deep breath and locked the car, the warmth of the sun delicately arousing my senses as I strode with a purpose to the reception entrance that loomed ahead. I had to walk past the first bay window and saw that it was full of people. A meeting seemed to be taking place and I held my head high, targeting the reception desk. "Can I help you?" a lady greeted me with an enquiring glance.

"I have a meeting at 2pm with the Chief Executive," I replied calmly.

"Can you please sign the visitors' book?" It was an order rather than a request and I nervously picked up the pen and scribbled the details down. "If you would take the next door to the right, I am sure he won't be long." She had already turned to continue her work, and I walked hesitantly to the door she had mentioned. The room was quite bare. It had a drinking water facility in one corner and a table. It was separated from the reception by special glass glazing and I scanned the rest of the room. A whiteboard detailing the meetings and timetables hung on the left wall, and in the middle of the table were several leaflets about the NHS Trust. Artwork from some of the patients decorated the walls.

Thirty minutes later I was still clock-watching when the door opened and a middle-aged gentleman walked in. "Hello, sorry I am late. The meeting went on longer than expected." His smile was genuine and he extended his hand. I shook it, rising to my feet, and I pulled my coat back on and followed him down the corridor to the left into his room, the one with the first bay window. A big round table stood in front and he beckoned me to take a seat. He explained to me why he liked a round table, and I felt like searching the room for Excalibur. I smiled as he continued to talk. "It is as if I know you already after reading your book."

I laughed back. "I hope that's a good thing, then," I replied, smiling. It was his turn to laugh again, and I leaned back feeling a bit more relaxed than I had done earlier. The conversation went better than expected, and I warmed to him. Antony, as he told me to call him, offered me a drink but I declined and he also admitted that he was pushed for time as he had to be in Nottingham in a short while. He told me that if we didn't get through all the issues, he would be happy to see me again. We did manage to discuss my time in the psychiatric ward, and I also mentioned how I thought a feedback system could be a potential idea on the nurses. I was still shocked at how some people were allowed to keep their jobs as nurses when it was so clear that they didn't care at all about the patients and saw their position as a power trip. At the same time other nurses were so brilliant at their jobs that they seemed to be underestimated by all. I thought a feedback system would work if it operated in a particular way. During my time on the wards I had little to do but observe.

***

Flashback:
It was around 7pm and I walked down the corridor of the ward to the reception area. I was not alone being on level one, and the agency nurse who was with me was laughing and chatting. "Don't worry, I'll ask her. I can't see why we can't go out." I shook my head as I knew who was in charge this evening and the words 'power trip' came into my mind before she even came into my sight.
She was there: a small figure standing in the crowded reception area. The patients had started to queue for their medicines. The trolley stood back in the small medical room, and as we approached she shouted out, "If you are going out, watch her. She is an opportunist and will misbehave at the slightest chance. Don't trust her and don't stand for any nonsense." The ward had gone silent and as I felt every pair of eyes in the room on me, I quickened my pace and walked through the double doors down the corridor to the exit. "You behave yourself, do you hear!" she was shouting down the corridor, her voice echoing off the walls. "Are you OK?" My agency nurse looked concerned and very angry. I was actually shaking inside, yet still wanted to go out

so I smiled, nodding. "I am fine and actually if you ask any other nurse you will find that I have never ran off when I have gone out for a walk. Dr Lynn trusts me and I would not break that trust. Walking around outside actually helps me and I would not want to risk losing that privilege. She talks as if I cause trouble on purpose, but I don't. I do act out but usually when I am panicking and that is usually because I feel trapped or have been working through things. Outside that is less likely to happen." My nurse was nodding her head and she patted me on the shoulder as if to give me some reassurance. "You could put in a complaint about her."

"It wouldn't get me anywhere, and if anything she would probably even treat me worse, if that is possible. I know that it is not me with the problem. I have watched her and she will be the first one to sit down whilst all the rest is working. She is always busy if anyone wants to talk, busy sitting and chatting. She sits back and watches the other nurses work, and believe me I get off lightly, although she does treat some of the male patients nicely." I suddenly went quiet as I didn't like to disrespect anyone and my nurse had gone quiet. I knew it would be unprofessional for her to comment back, and we both walked on in silence.

***

As I chatted to Antony about how I thought the feedback proposal would be a good idea, the incident of where the nurse picked on me verbally in front of everyone stuck in my mind. It hadn't been a major incident, but it had humiliated me and made me feel like a criminal. Some of the patients had jeered and clapped as because I was on level one some patients thought I was trouble, but in these patients' minds it was credible to be trouble. Another nurse had traumatised me when I was first admitted: she shouted and showed me up in front of everyone because I had innocently sat at a desk that I had been asked to sit at to build my confidence up. This nurse could have whispered to me that she didn't want me to sit there, but instead had been very rude and unprofessional. I had ended up running to my room and had started to cut myself. It was through sheer panic, and then this nurse had come in and had shouted even harder, threatening me with seclusion. She had been demanding if I *wanted* to be sent to seclusion. I had said I didn't know what seclusion was, and thought she was going to attack me. She got so angry, calling me a liar. I had only just come onto the unit and it was the first time in my life, and I hadn't got a clue what she was going on about. Then a junior doctor was sent to see me, and instead of being sympathetic I was told off and made to feel I was in the wrong. As I mentioned the feedback system, another nurse stuck in my head…

***

Flashback:
I nicknamed him 'The Walrus' because of his moustache. He liked to be in charge and I had first met him when he came into my room not long after I had been admitted and wanted to weigh me. He had seemed pleasant enough at the initial meeting, but it was later on when he had come into my room to take me to the patient assessment on ward round that I had first found out what he really like.

There was a short knock on the door and Lee entered. "Come on, time for ward round." I stared and was adamant that I was not going anywhere where I didn't know who was there and what it was for. "I'm not going."

"Don't be so silly. Come on."

I stayed put on my bed. "Get off that bed and come on. They are all waiting. You can't keep them waiting." His response was harsh and unpleasant. I stayed still and he went out briskly and very cross.

It was in the next hour that Dr Lynn had decided to come into my room with his junior doctor, and Lee had followed. With all these people entering my room at once, I had panicked and sprinted off the bed and out of the room. I was running hard when someone grabbed me around the waist and I desperately clawed at anything to get away. In the distance I could hear Dr Lynn calling me, and suddenly I stopped and looked round. I had been trying to claw my way through a brick wall and Karen one of the nurses had grabbed me around the waist. Dr Lynn told everyone to get out and he slowly took me back to my room. He had then let me miss the ward round assessment, coming in to see me privately. I was the only patient who was allowed to be absent, and I am sure Lee took a dislike to me for this. It was downhill from then on and I learned the meaning of cruelty.

***

I felt a need to add this unexpected paragraph. Rebecca, who is editing this book, made the following comment."As a reader, having been given a glimmer of what you had been through before this point, you do think 'what? Only now you learn the meaning of cruelty?!'. I don't know what this observation is worth, but it did really strike me!"

This feedback actually hit me and gave me insight about myself. I stand by what I wrote, as it truly felt that I was only learning the meaning of cruelty when I was in hospital with this particular nurse. At the same time I realise how ludicrous this can sound with relation to my past experiences. Although I can accept that what happened to me in my younger days would be seen as cruel from a reader's perspective, I think because I had no emotions that surfaced hitting me and hurting me as many were still suppressed, I hadn't at

88

that stage accepted the past. Some professionals may call it transference, as I was transferring or projecting my true feelings from the past into my present-day situation. I would deny that, as the incidents in the hospital tore me to pieces. I missed my children. This is another example of how denial and suppression play a huge part in child abuse consequences and trauma.

***

Lee would tell me I had to go through to the lounge to eat like the rest of the patients, even though he knew I had been given permission to eat in my room. I would have to argue and remind him. He constantly told me that I shouldn't be in hospital, that I was a time waster and should be home with my children. This upset me so much. I was sectioned and wasn't allowed out of the hospital. I was missing my children so much, and to have a staff nurse repeatedly tell you that you are a troublemaker and shouldn't be there caused pain that I didn't know existed. One evening he came into my room and went on so much that I tried to run out. He of course stopped me and told me to go back to my room. He then went on to tell me that I should be at home. I ended up self-harming and gave myself the biggest black eyes, and being upset marched out to aim for home. I then had two of the nurses hold me back as he was still shouting at me down the corridor. "Don't give him the satisfaction," Alex whispered. "Please, Bridge, he isn't worth it." I would not sit down, as Lee had managed to work me up so much. It was hell not seeing my kids and for him to tell me I should be at home and there was nothing wrong with me hurt so much. Then Lee started shouting that he was sending me to seclusion for not sitting down when told. It was at that point I rang Joseph and asked him to come. Joseph came as soon as possible. He looked anxious and was upset when he saw my face and very angry. He told me he had been to see Lee and had asked him if he knew why I was there. Apparently Lee had told him that he didn't as he hadn't bothered to look at my file. Joseph wanted me to leave, but we both knew I couldn't as I was sectioned. It was to be a long night and Joseph was worried sick as he eventually left me to return home to look after the children.

***

As I talked to Antony about my proposals for a feedback system, I was thinking mainly of these two nurses. There were others, but it was these two that stuck in my head. The other nurses were a male from a neighbouring ward who handled me roughly when I had escaped and called me a bitch and a whore. He had sworn repeatedly, and at another time when I had been really ill and had escaped through a top window that was unsecure because of

89

a broken catch. I was up at the top of a ladder being guided down by firemen when this nurse who was at the window had verbally mouthed 'bitch' at me and I had climbed back up.

It was him and another nurse who had used the restraining hold, but had brutally bent my wrist back so much that I fell on the floor in pain on the way to the seclusion room. My wrist suffered pains for the next year or so. The other nurse who had scared me was not through physical force: she was a nurse from the agency and would continually tell me that the devil was waiting for me. She would tell me that I had to pray for forgiveness, to pray to be a good mother and that I should go to church. She freaked me out, and on one occasion after the staff had promised they wouldn't hire her again she was on the rota to look after me again. I escaped on purpose with the help of a nurse who thought I had reason to go. Paula, who still is a great friend, arranged to meet me and she put me up at her house for the night. She had rung the ward to let them know I was OK. The ward had not been pleased, but I still believe today that they were in the wrong.

As I spoke to Antony, I felt the passion and conviction of my reasoning because of my past experiences.

"The only problem you have with feedback is the Erickson theory of In Group and Outer Group." I paused, as there were so many points to be made. "The staff will cover up for their own, and even the staff who are caring and professional will cover for the bad nurses. The patients will group up as well. A feedback system will work if it is handled professionally and systematically."

Antony was nodding and agreeing. I told him about how some of the elderly patients had been mismanaged, and that even some of the staff had asked me to feed back to them discreetly about night-time activities. I was in a great position to do this as my room was opposite the ladies' dormitory and I could see as well as hear about what went on in some cases. I was so worked up on this one, as I related some of the elderly ladies to my nan, and I loved my nan so much. One old lady would call out every night-time as she needed help with her toilet requirements. One set of nurses who happened to work together quite a lot would ignore her and then tell her to be quiet, and then be rough with her so she cried out. This upset me to such an extent that I was willing to spill the beans, and it took me all my willpower not to get involved at the time of the incidents.

Antony was listening intently and I tried to use the session constructively. I hadn't just gone there to moan. I sang the praises of the nurses who were so professional and caring. I wasn't biased in any form; I just told it as I had seen it. The session had to wind up, as the time passed quickly. Antony asked if I would visit the new ladies' acute ward to see what I thought of it.

He also praised my book as he thought the insight was significant. I was cheeky and asked if it was possible for him to write an endorsement, and to my delight he agreed.

***

I had walked away from the meeting with new hope. There was just a new glimmer of light that someone higher up in authority did care about what was happening in the local NHS Partnership Trust. I suppose there might have been others that did, but I had not been given that impression. Antony had impressed me, and it wasn't to do with him being the CEO of the local NHS Trust. It was because he was a down-to-earth, genuine man who was passionate about his job, passionate about the care, and working hard to fight for people who needed the care the Trust gave. I thought that the more people like that in authority, the more likely improvement would be made in the end.

***

CHAPTER TWELVE – THE RABBIT WARREN

Shit, shit, shit. I wasn't saying it, but I was thinking it. I rarely swore out loud but I was thinking *shit* as I pulled up in the car park. Why did I agree? Would I have a flashback? Would I embarrass myself?

My heart was beating rapidly as I locked my car and looked for the entrance to the ladies' acute ward. I walked down the back of the building. Walking down the narrow lane, I stopped in my tracks as I realised this was the lane where they brought me when I was admitted to the high security unit a few years back. When I had been admitted, the ambulance had stopped near the door and I had been rushed inside through one door and stopped before I was allowed to enter the main unit. Now, as I stood outside free, I was taken back by the building. The significance seemed to have evaporated: the building looked older, smaller and unimportant. I felt emotional as that was the time I should have been on a plane to Disneyland with my family, and instead I was rushed to this place. I also felt bitter because I had been brought up to believe Disneyland was a magical place and I had to live with the memory of my husband and kids flying there without me. Even now, the photos of their break pulls at my heartstrings. Joseph had booked it as a surprise whilst I was in hospital. I knew that I was too ill to go, and so did Joanie, my friend and neighbour. My consultant at the time had good-hearted intentions to allow me a break, yet he hadn't realised how it scared and freaked me out. I had tried to tell him, but he wanted me to have this holiday and enjoy myself. The thought of going away from hospital when I had been nearly institutionalised and on continuous level ones scared the daylights out of me. It scared me so much that the moment I was free, I had irrationally bolted for the nearest exit. It had happened to be on the second storey up, where a window had a broken catch, and looking round panicking, it had pulled me. All the other windows were locked and I grabbed the chance to get free. I wasn't thinking rationally, as the doors were not locked and really I could have just walked away. I think because I had been under supervision and restrained for so long, the first freedom was the first route I saw. I think if all the windows had been opened I wouldn't have been attracted to this route. It was because this was a broken catch and an unexpected route to freedom that I took it. I jumped out of the window onto a very narrow ledge on the top. This eventually led to me being detained in this high security unit, which as I looked at it now just brought a sick feeling inside. The first warning I was given when I entered was, "You don't have sheets. You have to earn your bed sheets." The man had told me this very sternly. I shivered and turned away from the building and looked for the entrance to the ladies' ward.

The nurse in charge welcomed me and I followed her from the main reception to the ward. It wasn't straightforward, and I felt like I was in a rabbit warren, and wondered if I would find my way out. The staff nurse was friendly and she told me she had read my book and enjoyed it.

She warned me that the ward was new so that all the facilities would not be in place, and I just thanked her for letting me visit. I felt nervous and tried hard not to show it.

We entered the double doors. "To the right we have the canteen area." She beckoned with her arm and I looked. "Here we will have my office. I am still putting everything in place." We walked into a double room on the left and she took me through to the room at the back where her desk was. She was very friendly and polite and I accepted the offer of a cup of tea.

The new ward was supposed to be much nicer because there were ten single rooms for the women, each with their own toilet and sink. I was taken back by how quiet it was, and I wondered if because there was less social contact than on a dormitory that was the reason why. We walked around and I automatically searched for danger zones. By this I mean ways to self-harm, ways to escape and places to hide. I immediately spotted a wooden chair in the quiet room. The quiet room was where you could go to relax, be on your own and wind down. I suppose you could do this to some extent in your own room, but this room was specifically designed for this purpose. There was nothing in it except for a sofa and a wooden chair. I immediately thought the chair was dangerous and the staff nurse, as if she'd read my mind, said, "That chair shouldn't be in here. It will be coming out." I also noticed five double-socket power points on the wall, and to me this seemed ludicrous as this room was supposed to be a safe room if someone felt bad. I didn't say anything then, but in my mind when there was nothing in the room except for the sofa you automatically were drawn to these sockets. Dangerous, I thought.

A normal dining chair with wooden arm rests would not seem unsafe to most people, yet having been a patient and having some insight I knew that it could be used in various ways to self-harm. When you are detained in a psychiatric hospital, or even in any other environment where you are out of your normal surroundings and possibly detained, then the context and environment can change your thinking dramatically, coupled with the fact that a person could be vulnerable and not thinking straight. I also understood that some patients were severely depressed and needed to self- harm and when everything is restricted to make it safe they can go to extremes to use anything possible. This stretches the mind to facilitate the use of items that would normally be thought of as safe. When you are on a diet, you immediately crave what you cannot have, and restrictions were met with demands.

***

I thought back to the first day of my admittance in the local ward. I was placed on a ward with mostly old people and in a room on my own. I was shy – so shy that I was restricted to a small area containing a bed, a wardrobe and a sink. I was too restless to read, and I was not a person to sit down doing nothing. I could not even spend time making a drink or something to eat, and within minutes I was bored. I still had a plate and a knife from my meal. I picked up the knife and started to unscrew the door-handle plate and other items that I could see. I was not intending to damage anything; I just needed to be occupied and I was a practical person. This meant I was busy.

Dr Lynn chuckled when he saw the room and the ward secretary at the time was nice about it. They wouldn't let me put the items back in place, saying they had to use the person whose job it was for maintenance. I think I kept him in work that summer.

***

At the new ladies' ward the staff nurse was pleasant and she took me back to her room for a chat. I couldn't understand it being at the back where she couldn't see any action. I thought if I wanted to manage a ward, I would want a room in the centre to be able to know what was happening. Yet there could be many reasons she chose the back room, possibly to get more work done without being disturbed, or she may have had a more laidback approach and was confident her staff could manage whilst she was busy. Anyway, she was very nice and approachable. I was quite forthright and did ask her that if I had to take any message back from her to Antony about the ward, what would it be. She was honest and replied that she was disappointed that at that time the ward wasn't being used for the full potential it was built for. She went on to explain, "Instead of having the women who needed the specialised support, where we can help and identify their problems and help them work through them, at the moment we are taking on patients on a postcode system and because we have spaces available. This means that the work I thought I was going to do isn't happening at the moment." She smiled ruefully and I felt for her, as it was obvious that the ward was caught up in the system, which depended on and was run by the availability of resources. Just then one of her nurses came running in. He looked like a rabbit caught in headlamps. "Sorry, we need you urgently." She had already got to her feet and she sent me an apologetic look as she ran after him. She had warned me at the beginning that emergencies might crop up and I had already realised this. I watched as they helped a young girl, possibly in her twenties, get up from the floor, and the staff nurse guided her into the medical room. I could tell by the trail of blood that she had managed to self-harm, and my heart went out to her. I knew that could have been me a while back. I took the opportunity to walk around the place. It was light and airy, and as I walked down the corridor it opened out wider and there was a little glass room in the centre where the staff worked. To the right there was the quiet room and another room where they were going to have some computers. The doors to the dormitory stayed closed, and apart from one patient with another lady who I presumed to be her mother, the ward seemed quiet. The odd member of staff walked by me, and while some acknowledged me with a smile, some did not look up. The ward seemed bare, with just a couple of plants stood on the odd table. I looked around, and there was a television in one room. I could see no books or activities to do, and it reminded me of a dentist's waiting room with the odd magazine spread about. I took a deep breath and was so glad I was leaving shortly. The building was much better, as it was new and light instead of dark and dismal, yet the atmosphere was nearly non-existent.

Twenty minutes later, the staff nurse appeared. The young girl had her arm bandaged up and had gone back to her room. I followed her back for a quick chat before I left. She explained that because the ward was so new, the activities they had planned for hadn't yet been put into place and more resources like books and games were on their way. She did take me outside to the grass area at the back and I surveyed the metal fencing and decided I would not have been able to get out from there. We both decided it was still quiet as it was only ten o clock in the morning, but I still felt that the old wards would have been bustling. I came away with mixed feelings: I was glad I had been given the chance to look around, and felt privileged she had taken time out to see me, but I hadn't liked the atmosphere in there. I hoped that my snapshot was just a snapshot, and that at other times it would have had more life and colour in the place, not just a clinical silver and white with the odd splash of blood.

***

On my return I sent Antony an email informing him that I had been to visit the new ward, and I was dismayed as I just received an acknowledgement back thanking me without any question of feedback. This upset me, and although I know I should have the deepest respect that Antony had even bothered to see me, I was annoyed that I had stepped up to the challenge of seeing the ward because I thought my feedback was valuable. I didn't sit on it: I replied back and conveyed these exact thoughts. The following week I received another invitation to meet Antony.

I was pleased to receive the letter, but I also felt nervous as I was returning to a meeting where I had complained about how I had been treated. I prefer to lay my cards out on the table, and with this meeting I did that. I still massively appreciated the time that Antony had given to me previously, and that he had responded to my grievances and was still seeing me. The meeting went very well, and if anything it strengthened my respect and admiration for the Chief Executive of the local Trust. He listened carefully and he took the time to explain the different issues. I conveyed the staff nurse's thoughts, and I left feeling reassured that he was doing his best to carry out an enormously difficult job with so much pressure, and that the most important thing of all was that he cared about what happened to not only the patients in his care but the whole mental health system.

***

CHAPTER THIRTEEN – REMEMBRANCE DAY

The days were drawing in and it was chilly in the evenings. I now had to put the hens away as it was too late by the time Tee Jay arrived home. We were lucky because we had booked for some decorators to paint the outside of the house and the weather, although misty and damp first thing in the morning, cleared into nice days. There was only one day when they had to go home early due to rain.

Asti, our schnauzer, would jump and bark at strangers. She was loving, but very protective. Amba was a massive softy and would greet anyone with what little she had of a tail wagging like mad. She would also answer back, and if anyone spoke to her she would go into a soft singsong of a bark. People would laugh and this would please her and she would do it more. She was a gentle giant and I loved her so much. She seemed to understand my moods, and if I was having an off day she would walk up to me and place her nose into my hands and push up. I would then give her a huge hug and I think we comforted each other. She would then go into her singsong of a bark and it would motivate me to get up and fetch her a biscuit or play with her. She was growing old, and if I threw the ball Asti would usually get there first and then show off with it. Amba didn't mind; I reckon she was secretly pleased she didn't have to fetch it. She was losing her eyesight and it reminded me that she was getting on. She was twelve and a half, and Gina, my last Italian Spinone, had lived to fourteen and a half so I hoped Amba would do the same.

Today was Thursday November 10th 2011, and I decided to strip and make our bed as it was such a nice day. The decorators had started rubbing down the woodwork, and I could hear Amba answering one of them back from her kennel as he painted the window next to her. I could hear him laughing at her. I changed my attention to the bed and went to the bathroom to pick the bed linen from the cupboard. As my hand reached out and touched the linen, I remembered…

Flashback:

"We had better go and pick your sheets out," said Karen, my level one nurse. I followed her down to the end of the corridor where she unlocked a door to the right and beckoned me in. She started to grab a sheet from the big pile on the shelf in the cupboard. I went to take it from her. "No." She grabbed it back. "Look at it first." Her big eyes rolled up to the ceiling and back at me. I shrugged my shoulders. I was new at this and didn't know what to expect. As she held the sheet out I initially felt like vomiting for there near the top were some greenish marks, and what was worse was that they were lumpy. I grimaced, and she laughed. "Don't worry, there will be some better than others. They have all been laundered, but some stuff still doesn't wash off." We went through the next few sheets and the sixth one was fine. I inspected the pillowcases: the same, and Karen laughed as I even turned them inside out. The nurses were nice to me and I was lucky that I could pick my own sheets, and I also picked some extra blankets as one of the nurses had told me to place one on the bottom of the bed under the sheet. The nurses were kind and often if it was chilly at night would help me with the bed linen. It was unpleasant to find out that the sheets were like they were, yet months later I didn't think anything of it. It became a natural routine to take time to pick the cleanest ones out.

***

I finished making our beds and went downstairs to make the decorators a drink of tea. The sun was shining and they were on schedule. We were all happy as they predicted they would be finished by early afternoon. I went inside to play with the kittens. We had decided to keep five out of the eight. Our neighbour was having the long-haired ginger, who they named Tsar, and the short-haired tortoiseshell Molly. She was lovely, but was always the kitten who had escaped or who had been naughty. Tsar was beautiful in looks and Molly was playful in character. My friend Gail also had the tiniest ginger and white kitten. Her daughter named him Garfield. She took him to bed with her every night, and it was nice for Tee Jay as he could ask her at school how Garfield was doing.

I loved all the cats, and had initially thought Gail would also have Batman, a little black and white cat with white socks who snuggled up to anyone who would have him. He was cute being the smallest, and he had massive ears like bats and was so active. Gail eventually decided only on Garfield and I was happy as I had a soft spot for Batman. Joseph always liked ginger cats, and he had told me he wanted to keep Tiger, so-called because of his markings. Tee Jay wanted to keep Rolo, a long-haired tortoiseshell who loved to roll over and followed Tee Jay everywhere. I had picked Muffin, another long-haired cat; he reminded me of the black and white cat in the *Postman Pat* stories. This only left Ninja, so-called because he acted tough yet was a phoney, being the softest cat of them all. He was similar to Garfield and had pale ginger and white markings. He never stopped purring and Jo Jo had picked him.

Now, as the sun shone and the decorators were painting the finishing touches, I rolled the ball and all five kittens chased it. Rolo won and swiped it across the room. I laughed as the mob went chasing after it again. Bella had disappeared out for some fresh air. Petrus, our old cat, looked on with interest. I was wary as I walked around the house, as I never knew which window the decorators would pop up at. They were doing a good job and the dark woodwork gleamed new life into the building. I laughed as I could hear Amba answering back again to one of the men. She was lazing in her kennel whilst Asti kept pacing. I washed the pots and went outside to inspect the house as they were packing away. "Excellent," I remarked to Lionel as he showed me around. I paid their bill and thanked them as they left.

The next day was Remembrance Day, and I was browsing through Facebook looking at the different poppy pictures that people had posted on their profiles. I glanced at the time: it was around eleven o'clock, and I wondered if I had missed the minute's silence on the television. Asti jumped up at my patio door and I stared outside, thinking I hadn't seen Amba this morning. As I walked outside towards her kennel, I could see her nose just peeping out, resting on her paws. "You lazy girl," I joked as I bent down to greet her. It was then that my world seemed to fall apart in a split second. Amba wasn't moving, and in disbelief I reached out and touched her. She was stone cold. I sank to my knees and hugged her, feeling guilty that I hadn't been there for her, guilty that I hadn't noticed anything wrong, an awful dread of a loss tore at my heart. I stared at her. She just looked like she had fallen asleep with her head resting on her paws. I hoped that she had gone peacefully in her sleep. I walked slowly indoors and I suddenly felt such an intense despair it frightened me.

I rang my doctor up as I was panicking. I felt like I wanted to smash the place up but felt calm at the same time. Julie the receptionist answered, and I said, "Hi". She recognised me straightaway.

"Hi, Dr Dhanji is away."

"Oh I forgot, and Maggie is away too, isn't she?" I stated as I remembered. "Don't worry. I just found my dog has died in her kennel and I am in a bit of a state."

"Oh, that's awful. I am sorry," said Julie. She continued to talk at random to me, trying to reassure and comfort me, and I was grateful as it was giving me time to compose myself whilst at the same time having a safe contact at hand. I interrupted when I felt calmer. "Thanks, Julie. I shall have to go in case someone is trying to get through to your surgery." I placed the phone down thankful that my doctor had such a nice receptionist. I sat down and realised that I felt everything was surreal and just stared at the wall.

I still felt numb so I rang my mum up. The phone rang a few times and I knew she struggled to get to it. "Hi Mum, are you free a minute?"

"No, not really. The hairdresser will be here in a second," Mum replied. "Why?"

"Don't worry, I've just lost Amba. She is dead in her kennel." I heard the gasp and my mum panicking.

"Are you sure you are alright? I am so sorry, darling. Do you want me to come up?"

"No, Mum. Thanks, but you can't do anything. I'll be fine. It is still a shock."

"Don't do anything stupid. You'll be alright?"

"Mum, I promise. I'll be fine."

"I'll ring you later."

"OK, Mum. I love you." I placed the phone down and sank against the wall. I felt sick and numb and I thought I ought to ring Joseph, as I reckoned he would be at the shop by now.

"Hello?" his voice was questioning.

"Hi, I have some bad news." My voice was faltering. I knew I was cracking up again.

"What?" he sounded concerned.

"We've lost Amba. I've just found her in the kennel."

"Oh, poor girl," he said quietly. "Well, I can't come back and I can't do anything about it."

His response irritated me. "No, we'll just leave her there," I replied.

There was a silence. "Do you want me to come back and bury her?"

"No." I was adamant as I knew he would do something wrong. Joseph was very accident-prone. I could picture him not digging the grave deep enough, and I knew she was too big. I also wanted her to have dignity.

"No, leave it. The children may want to say goodbye. I am fine. Just let me think." I sighed and placed the phone down. I walked into the kitchen and again I felt such an extreme intensity that it scared me. It was similar to the intense feelings when I wanted to self-harm or be suicidal. I didn't want to believe this was happening. I rang Joanie, my friend and neighbour, and she answered her mobile straightaway.

"What are you doing? Can you come round?"

"Why, what's up? I'm on my way." She could sense the desperation in my voice, and minutes later she was knocking at my door. I opened it, and taking one look at her I crumpled against the wall, still standing but only just.

"What on earth has happened? You look awful. What is it?" Joanie looked concerned and I had a job to answer.

100

"She's dead, in the kennel. I just found her." My voice had gone up a few pitches. My fingers scraped the wall. I stared but I was staring out. I was staring away.

"Who's dead? Who is in the kennel?" Joanie's voice now had an urgent sound.

"Amba," I whispered.

"Oh no, how? Oh no." Joanie looked shocked. "When?"

"About eleven this morning. I won't forget the time or the date."

"Tea with loads of sugar." Joanie started marching me to the kitchen.

"Don't forget I am diabetic now. I am on insulin," I muttered.

"Oh shit, I'll end up killing you either way." Joanie joked that she was never very good with my sugar control.

She made me a tea without sugar whilst she had a coffee.

"Do you want Martin to bury her?"

Nodding, I sipped my tea slowly. "Please could he do it later, as the children may want to say goodbye. Do you think he would bury her around the lakes where we spent a lot of time together?" Amba loved going on walks around the lakes.

"I am sure he will," smiled Joanie. I smiled back and she sat with me for a while and then said she had to go as Claire would be missing her. "Thanks, as always," I muttered.

It was just after she had gone that a car pulled up in the driveway. My heart lurched as I looked out of the window. An elderly lady was struggling to get out of the car.

"Mum." I was so pleased to see her, yet so concerned that she had driven knowing it would have caused her pain because of her hip replacement.

We stood and hugged each other in silence and Mum turned to me. "I had to come." I nodded. She made to go out through the back.

"Mum, please don't go out there." I had just gained some strength and knew I couldn't face Amba yet. My mum sat and had a cup of tea and a biscuit, and although she meant well it added to my anxiety. She hadn't been here long, and already the sun was starting to go down. "Mum, I don't want you to go but you must. The sun is setting, and I know you have a job to see with the glare. I want you home safe before it gets too strong."

My mum got to her feet and again hugged me. "Are you sure you will be OK?"

I nodded and hugged her back. It meant so much to me that she had made the effort to drive over, and I was anxious that she return safely. I walked to the door with her, and reversed her car out of the drive for her. She hooted the horn as she left, and I smiled and waved at the disappearing vehicle. I returned to the kitchen and looked at the clock: the kids would be home in ten minutes, another reason why I wanted Mum out of the way. It was going to be so tough telling my children that their beloved Amba had died. I paced and paced until I heard them come through. They were laughing and teasing each other.

They entered the kitchen, and Tee Jay flung his coat on the table, Jo Jo following him. I didn't waste time. Walking up, I placed my arms around both of them. "I need you to come into the lounge. I have some very bad news." They followed me and I knew from the look on their faces that they knew it was serious.

"We've lost Amba." I could say it no easy way.

"No!" Jo Jo nearly screamed and immediately started to cry. Tee Jay broke down and the two just sobbed cuddling up to me. "How?" Jo Jo sniffled.

"I found her this morning in her kennel. It looks like she died peacefully in her sleep. She may not have known anything about it." Both the children set off again, and I stared miserably into the air, at a loss as to how to console them. I thought rationally, but before I could say anything Jo Jo asked, "Can we see her?" I sat her down and looked into her eyes.

"Are you sure you want to? It may upset you. Martin is coming soon and he is going to bury her in a nice place around the lakes."

Jo Jo had already got up. "I want to see her." She started to walk outside and Tee Jay hesitantly followed. Jo Jo bent down and started to stroke Amba on the head, straightening her fur. I looked on with tears in my eyes. She then bent over and kissed her on the head. "Bye bye, girl. You were one of the best." She walked away crying, and I wanted to follow, but Tee Jay now stroked her and gave her a kiss. He was silent but I knew he was upset. "You two have to be specially nice to Asti, as she is really moping," I said, hoping it would give them direction.

Martin and Mick pulled up outside the house, bringing in a big blanket. I posted the sad news on Facebook, and Jo Jo posted a very moving message with a photograph of Amba that made me feel proud of how loving my daughter could be.

In the following weeks our attention turned to Asti because she was moping badly, and had started to steal any soft toy that she could find. She also started to nurse the kittens. Several times she went into the kennel and started to whimper. It upset me and I called her over. "Asti, come on, girl." She would run up, and I hugged her tightly.

I missed Amba, and I knew I had to look for another Spinone quickly to help us all recover and to give Asti a new playmate. I knew Amba could never be replaced, and just hoped that I could find another Italian Spinone that could again give us so much joy.

CHAPTER FOURTEEN – CHRISTMAS 2011

It was coming towards the end of November and I was nervous. I searched the internet for my Open University home page every day, and each time I looked I felt sick clicking the link to see if any results were in and had butterflies in my stomach. Today I didn't have time to feel sick because as soon as I opened my student home page I had a message saying, 'Congratulations, you have achieved a First Class (1.1) Honours Psychology degree.' I felt elated and excited. I ran upstairs to the office to tell Joseph.

"Guess what?" I laughed, and ran and jumped on his knee.

"You've passed!" He grinned as his office chair spun round with us both on it.

"First class honours," I said proudly.

"Well done. I always knew you could do it." He gave me a kiss and a hug, and I jumped up, as I wanted to ring my mum up.

"Mum, guess what? I've done it, I got the first class honours."

"Oh darling, I am so proud of you! I wish your dad was alive to hear this." My mum was so happy.

"He knows, Mum. Every exam I used his pen and told him to wish me luck." I heard my mum take a deep breath. I could tell she was happy but sad that my dad couldn't have been here.

"You deserve it, darling. You worked so hard for that."

"I tried my hardest, Mum. That's all I could do." I laughed and I nearly felt like crying as after all these years I had done it and achieved my goal. I proved all those wrong that had said because I hadn't had a higher education I would not be able to achieve a first. I had proved to myself that I was worthy of gaining a first and that if you believed in yourself with perseverance and hard work you could achieve your dreams.

"Bye, Mum. I love you."

"Love you too, darling. Congratulations," Mum said.

I placed the phone down and I rang Maggie, my diabetic nurse who had wished me luck all the way.

"Mags, I did it. I got my first."

"I knew you would," she replied. "Can you go on and study diabetes?"

We both laughed. I was so happy.

Maggie had supported me and wished me luck all the way. She too had told me off at times for expecting too much. She would tell me off and say anyone else would be happy for just passing. I knew deep down I would not have been happy for just passing as I was too competitive. I had set myself a target and it had kept me focused. Now, suddenly, I felt very lost. This target had kept me on track for seven years, and now I felt free. I knew that to keep myself safe I had to keep occupied 24/7, and this was because as soon as I had any free time my mind would become flooded with unwelcome memories. Flashbacks would cause distress and instability, and to keep memories at bay I needed to keep busy. My university degree had kept me occupied, but it had also meant that I had to sacrifice valuable family time and other quality time for me to finish my degree. I was lucky because Joseph, Jo Jo and Tee Jay supported me throughout. Some of my friends thought I was mad to do a degree and to write a second book, but many people had asked me to and I felt that the first had not included all I wanted it to.

People asked me how I remembered such detail, and I answered that the first book was on autopilot and it just streamed out. The dates may not have been exact, but the events were more or less in chronological order. This book was so much harder as the content was easier but I had to think about it. I didn't like thinking, and it was as if my mind had a protection lever. I could free-think, as I called it, and chat and respond to anything that came to mind. If I was questioned and the answer was easy I could manage easily. It was when I had to think or concentrate deeply about any subject that I had problems. It was as if my mind shut down and I could think no more.

I wasn't happy to be in this state, and I reflected and questioned why…

My answer to myself was that I guessed it was a coping strategy to keep anything that may be uncomfortable or dangerous to my mind at bay. I still suffered flashbacks, and although they were few and far between, they could be intense and frightening. I guessed that if my mind blocked off at a certain level then all it was doing was protecting me. It was frustrating when I tried to concentrate hard, as my speech would start to stutter and my head felt fuzzy. It was the same for conversations. I had a habit of breaking off mid-sentence if it was going too deep and changing the subject. This was all done unintentionally and had become a bad habit. My friends had become used to guessing the end of the sentence and sometimes laughed at the rapid change in direction of the topic.

Dr Dhanji was also pleased for me that I had achieved a first-class honours degree. It had become a joke the last few months, as I had been panicking every time I had gone to see her. My anxiety levels had risen and it seemed to have a knock-on effect as I panicked about every little detail: about Joseph, the kids and anything else that came my way. I had good reason to panic about our future, as with the recession biting deeper we were finding it hard to keep up with the mortgage payments. Joseph would tell me that with Christmas coming the business would pick up. Christmas was approaching, but the weather held out. The snow was not around nor was the business.

I also had to pay a deposit for my new puppy, and she didn't come cheap. The full sum made a big hole in our pockets. I justified it to myself as the whole family, including Asti, was still missing Amba. I still looked forward to Christmas, and I still spent more than I should have done. I loved Christmas Day, and I really looked forward to seeing the kids open their presents. I liked the carol-singing, the bell-ringing and the spirit of Christmas. I disliked it when shops started selling festivity items in July, and although I disliked the commercial entity, I loved the essence of Christmas and always hoped the snow would fall on Christmas Day. This year Christmas seemed to creep up unexpectedly, and when the first Sunday in December dawned we were not so excited about putting the Christmas tree up and all the decorations. I dreaded getting the dog stockings out. We had two stockings designed as puppies. We had faithfully filled each with dog treats for both Amba and Asti and both dogs would get so excited. When the kids started to open their presents, the dogs would be given their treats. We pulled the stockings out of the box with sadness, and as I hung them both up Jo Jo started to cry. I took a deep breath. "Amba would want you to be happy and remember all the good memories," I said softly to Jo Jo. She stormed out of the room and I knew my daughter well enough to know this wasn't the time to follow her. She needed some space.

I hung the other stockings up. We had one for the cats, and we even had a very tiny one that used to be for the hamster. I smiled to myself as I hung it up on the fender. Some people would mock us, but our pets were our family and we enjoyed spoiling them too.

The weeks passed quickly and Tee Jay approached me as he came in from school. "Hey, Mum, please can I go into town tomorrow night from school?" He looked at me with his big brown eyes. I laughed and tousled his long and curly hair. "Why?" I asked.

"Mum!"

It was a statement and he replied quite angrily, as if I shouldn't have asked. I shrugged my shoulders. "Alright, alright, yes you can, but don't take too much money to school."

"Mu-um."

I sighed and shrugged my shoulders. My son didn't like me giving advice to him anymore. The next day Tee Jay reminded me that he would need picking up later and that he would ring me when he was ready. Joseph and I had just about got used to being a taxi service, and with no bus route for two miles we were in huge demand. The lane near our house was a cut-through to the town, and with it only being a small lane with no pathways or pavement I was reluctant to let the kids walk along it. The traffic would speed, and there were often accidents with the hedgerows broken, and tyre skid marks across the road.

Once the kids were at school I decided to look through what I had bought them. The trouble was I bought things when I saw them, and often forgot what I had bought by the time Christmas drew near. I was satisfied that both Jo Jo and Tee Jay had about equal presents and I pondered what other gift I could buy Joseph. It was hard, as I was trying to save money and make sure if I did spend it was something he really wanted. All I ever got when I asked was the reply, "Nothing. I don't need anything." It wasn't helpful as he knew he would receive something and I needed to think hard what to get.

Tee Jay rang at about 5pm and I could tell he was excited. He waited for me in the local swimming pool car park.

He beckoned to me as I pulled in, a slight motion of the hand as if to say 'Here I am', but discreetly enough not to let other people know he was waving to his mum. He clambered into the car, placing some shopping bags on the back seat. "Don't look round, Mum."

I laughed. "I don't intend to. This car won't drive by itself," I retorted.

"Won't it?" He laughed, acting surprised. I laughed too.

"Had a good day?" I asked.

He nodded his head whilst reading the messages on his phone. "Is Jo Jo back?" he asked.

"Yes, she is doing some homework in her room," I replied.

"More likely she is on Facebook," he answered. I shrugged my shoulders as I drove onto our driveway. Tee Jay carried his bags upstairs and I went into the kitchen to make myself a cup of tea. Joseph was still out and I didn't expect him back until late evening. "Tee, don't forget to put the hens away!" I shouted. I started to make the dinner and was amused as eight of the cats decided to sit watching waiting for any titbit to fall. Gail had joked, "Be careful. You'll become known as the cat lady." She had ducked as I had thrown the nearest cushion at her.

Christmas Day came and we got up early and opened the presents from each other in the morning. Tee Jay had a new bicycle and I had to build it, so we made room in the lounge whilst Joseph started to prepare the Christmas dinner. "Pass the spanner, Mum. Thanks." I passed him the spanner.

"Not that way, darling. You're undoing it." Tee Jay laughed.

"I wondered why it wasn't getting tighter." He soon tightened the offending nut and started to tighten up the opposite side. Soon we had a spanking new bicycle ready to go. I followed him out through the front door and he rode up and down the lane. It was chilly and we came quickly inside to the warmth of the lounge and the delightful aroma of the turkey roasting.

Joseph brought some snacks through and we called Jo Jo down and watched the television whilst the dinner was cooking.

It was a quiet Christmas, as Mum was at my sister Denny's house and Joseph's parents were in Switzerland. The neighbours used to have parties, but some had gone away and gradually throughout the last years everyone had always seemed too busy to slow down and have a get-together. We all had good intentions, but never seemed to follow them through. Joanie was busy helping her daughter Claire prepare to train in a robotic suit to walk the London Marathon. If she managed to do it, then she would be the first person in the world with a broken back to complete the course in a robotic suit. It was a significant challenge, as they hadn't yet got the suit and no one was sure if it would be only a dream or if Claire would manage to achieve her goal. We sat in the kitchen pulling the crackers and telling the worst jokes. They were made even more comical with Joseph's accent and Tee Jay's mispronunciation.

We went for a walk on Boxing Day, and as we neared the lakes we remembered Amba as it was the first time we had walked as a family around there again without her. I searched for where her grave might be. Martin had told me roughly where it was, and I wanted to see it and yet I didn't. I scanned silently, as I didn't want to upset the kids and I am sure they were thinking about her too. The lakes were still and silent, the sky was grey and although dry it was calm except for the odd duck flying up startled as Asti ran by. We had walked around these lakes at this time of the year annually and never had we been so quiet as we were today.

The days passed quickly, and soon we were on our way to North Walsham in Norfolk to see the Italian Spinone puppies. We were excited. I was also anxious, hoping that I would be able to choose the one I liked. We were late as Joseph lost his way and we ended up in Norwich town on a Saturday afternoon.

Eventually we arrived and a warm welcome greeted us. As we sat in the lounge sipping our tea, our hosts Michael and Bibby brought Juno, the mother of the puppies, into the room. I immediately warmed to her, as she was so friendly. It was a change to see a chocolate roan, but she was a nice-looking dog and I already knew that I would love her puppies. We were also introduced to Basil, an orange and white Italian Spinone male. He was huge and very lovable. I had some fleeting thoughts in my mind whether I should have gone for an orange and white male, yet Asti was not neutered and I recognised it was my heart ruling my head just because he was an orange and white, but his nature was lovable. I missed Amba so much, and she was in the back of my mind all the time.

Michael and Bibby chattered to us, asking us questions, and I looked at the photo album of some of the Spinones Bibby had bred. We got on well, and the moment came when they invited us through to the back room to see the puppies. I was excited and apprehensive. It was such a big deal to me, and I knew that the choice I would make would affect us all as a family for the rest of our lives. Bibby and Michael had placed the males in a separate run to make it easier, and they also pointed out one of the puppies that had already been spoken for. Bibby said, "By the way, my little girl is the one in the basket. I think I'll be keeping her." My heart sank as I looked to the basket at the puppy with the very dark brown head that lay there. I had a soft spot for her from the photographs they had emailed previously. I immediately refused to look at her and concentrated on the rest of the puppies, who were all adorable. Jo Jo sat on the floor and fell in love with the smallest one called Misty. Michael interrupted and passed Drizzle, a chunkier looking puppy that reminded me of first Spinone Gina, to Joseph. As Joseph cuddled her, Tee Jay started playing with Gusty, who I also liked as she was very friendly. Gusty had already been chosen, and I started to try to pick the puppy I wanted. I was drawn to Drizzle, as she reminded me of Gina, and I liked the heavier, chunky look. Jo Jo said, "Which one, Mum?"

"I don't know." I shrugged my shoulders. Joseph turned round to look at me; he was standing on the outside of the pen, slightly reserved as he wasn't such a doggie person as I was. "I like this one. I think we should have this one." I smiled as he was pointing to Drizzle – without me saying he had picked the same puppy, which was so rare as we were usually so opposite in choice. "Yes, yes, Mummy," Jo Jo said, and as I looked at Tee Jay he was nodding. I picked Drizzle up, giving her a cuddle. "We've decided." I looked across to Bibby and smiled because I knew that I wanted this puppy. Bibby looked happy. "You will have to brush her a lot, as it looks like she will have a thick coat." I nodded. I didn't mind, and I was glad that we had managed to make a decision. Bibby and Michael asked us to make a second choice just in case, and with difficulty we did this. Bibby was pretty certain she was going to keep Breezy, the dark-headed one in the basket, "But they are only five weeks old and they can change, but I am pretty sure you will be safe with Drizzle."

Back at home I couldn't wait to post the news on my Facebook page and show off Drizzle, and within minutes people were posting positive comments about my new puppy. I started to let the excitement trickle through just a little. It was arranged with Michael and Bibby that we would pick up Drizzle on the Sunday before my birthday. A few days later we were all watching the television when the telephone rang. I could see by the number that it was Michael and Bibby. "Don't worry, I'll take it!" I shouted from across the hallway, and I ran through to my study room to chat with Bibby.

"So I am really sorry, but I have decided to keep Drizzle." My heart seemed to miss a beat, and I had an awful sinking feeling. I heard more apologies, and I tried my hardest to laugh it off, saying that I was so grateful to be having one of the puppies anyway. Later in the lounge I had to break the news to everyone and we were all upset. I went back to my study and looked again at the photographs of the puppies. It was then that it hit me: if Bibby was going to keep Drizzle, then the dark-headed puppy I had liked from the beginning...

I rang the number as quickly as I could. I was so nervous and yet so afraid that she too may have been taken. I spoke to Bibby and explained how I had loved this other puppy all the time and had not chosen her as I thought she wasn't available. "If you want Breezy then you shall have her. I felt so bad about Drizzle, as I could tell you were upset but still trying to be cheerful."

My emotions were all over the place and I was so happy. "Thank you, Bibby. I know you love her but I will look after her so well." I ran into the lounge. "Guess what? We're having Breezy!" The kids laughed and Joseph looked bemused. I nearly danced up the stairs to bed, and although I still felt sad about losing Drizzle I was so happy at gaining Breezy.

CHAPTER FIFTEEN – HOMECOMING

"What are we going to call her?" Jo Jo asked me again and I shrugged my shoulders. Every time I had come up with a name I liked, someone else didn't. I had tried to keep it Italian, and was now an expert on different types of pasta. We eventually managed to minimise our choice to two names: Tia and Cara.

Bibby passed Breezy to me with tears in her eyes. I held my new puppy tightly, enjoying the distinct aroma she gave out. I held her secure in a towel on my knee, making sure the seatbelt would protect both of us. Joseph drove carefully and slowed down a few times as Breezy was car-sick repeatedly. I cuddled her and changed the towelling repeatedly, and it was a relief to arrive home. Jo Jo and Tee Jay came running through and couldn't believe how much she had grown since we last saw her. "She has been ever so good," I said proudly, and watched her prance across the floor. Jo Jo laughed and after stroking her placed Breezy in the dog pen and we let Asti through. Both dogs started to sniff each other through the bars and I surveyed their body language. Asti was now wagging her tail and her ears were perked up more in amusement than anything else. Both were very excited and we let them get to know each other for a while.

We chose Cara for her name and much to our joy and amusement not only did Cara play with Asti but she was soon rolling around on the floor with the kittens. Bella and the older cats were not so sure, but the kittens ran to Cara for fuss and they soon became best friends.

My birthday came and went, and I was really happy to have Cara at home. She was mischievous and chewed everything and anything in sight. She learned how to play Joseph, and rolled over on her back if he raised his voice, with paws in the air. He ended up laughing more times than telling her off.

It was at this time that we started to receive many telephone calls, and Joseph would shout out to leave them. It worried me, as I knew we were struggling financially, and to have just bought a new puppy seemed frivolous, and yet my dogs were a huge part of my life. I did not socialise or spend money elsewhere, and in my mind I still justified buying Cara as Amba had left such a massive hole in our lives. It had not only affected us, as Asti had still been moping. Now with Cara she was like a young pup and they rolled and played together and Cara had brought a little sunshine back into our lives.

The telephone calls didn't go away, and the letters started to arrive, demanding settlements for our mortgage and other bills. Joseph started to try to get to the post before anyone else, and also to the phone. He became very stressed and started to shout at the smallest thing. I had no choice but to tackle him about our situation.

"How bad is it?" I looked directly into his eyes.

"I just need time," he said, and looked away. I felt cross as I didn't like to avoid the telephone calls and I wanted to face the problem. "It won't go away, you know. You need to do something about it and I am not asking you, I am telling you." Joseph looked at me and sighed. He shrugged his shoulders and walked away from me out of the room. I was in two minds whether to chase after him or leave him, but I decided to give him some space and hoped that he would take action.

"I'm going to talk to my supplier this morning to see if they will support me," Joseph stated as I sat on the sofa drinking my morning tea. I looked across at him and shrugged my shoulders. I was feeling frustrated, guilty that I hadn't any sympathy, and cross that he had left it this long. I sipped my tea in silence and got up to go and make the kids' sandwiches.

It was nearly midday when Joseph walked in. I heard the toilet flush and then the pounding of his footsteps going up to his office. It annoyed me he never came to say hello first, and I figured that if it had been good news he would have come straight in to tell me. I looked up my email messages and posted onto Facebook. My mind was elsewhere, and it was while I was putting the kettle on that he came into the kitchen.

"They have advised me to stop trading." He took a deep breath and looked at me. "I have booked an appointment with the bank manager and accountant."

"What are we going to do?" I asked with a sinking feeling.

"I don't know," Joseph said. He took the coffee I was offering him and we both stood in silence, sipping hot coffee and contemplating.

"Well, it's better you face up to it now, before it gets worse," I said. Joseph nodded, and taking the telephone walked out of the room. I went into my study. I felt sick and depressed. I decided that we should tackle the situation head-on and find out all of our options. It was to be a week later that Joseph had gathered the information we needed so that we could make an informed decision.

We both sat in the lounge and he worked out the debt. It was to be a lot worse than I thought, but the good part was that he had paid most of his suppliers. It was just a couple of big businesses that he owed money to, and I felt bad for them. I also felt bad for us, as because of his male pride he had tried to hide the debt from me and had borrowed stupidly. If we had talked we could have probably got a loan with a half-decent rate, but Joseph had taken the easiest options available to him and the most expensive. He had borrowed on his credit cards, and as I read the figures I felt sick. I got up and walked out of the room. Joseph came running after me and swung me around. "How could you?" I stared at him as I shook his arm away. "Don't touch me. You have lied to me, deceived me and now have borrowed ridiculously. If we were in that much trouble, why did you go skiing last year?"

My voice was raised, because I felt so sick knowing he had gone on an expensive skiing trip to St Anton all the time knowing we were in trouble. "Don't our kids come first?"

"I know, I know I shouldn't have gone. I couldn't help it." Joseph was pacing the room. "I didn't want you to know. I thought with time the situation would get better."

"You're stupid. You're an idiot. You lie, you cheat and I don't like you at this time." My voice had dropped and I looked away. "Come on, come here," Joseph pulled at my arm. I shook him off,

"No, you can't talk me around. To be honest I am upset we are in financial trouble, but I am more upset about the lies and the dishonesty. Why didn't you tell me? I could have looked for a loan. Why let it get this bad?" I sat down and stared at my computer without seeing it. "I can't trust you and what is our marriage worth if I can't trust you?" Joseph looked and shuffled his feet. I could tell he was uncomfortable.

"I have spoken to my brother and he is sure I could get a job in Switzerland and the money is so much better than here." It was my turn to look shocked, and I grabbed the chair for support. "I know you and the kids don't want to move, but I can go and get a job and visit at weekends or when I have time off. Even if we do it for two years I will have saved enough to get us out of this mess." Joseph walked up to me. I stood up and hugged him and he hugged me back. Arguing was one thing, but this was different. I didn't want him to go, but I also couldn't see a solution over here. Joseph's job was so specialised that unless he worked in London it would be difficult to find any other work. "There is something else," Joseph said, and he continued. "I have been advised to go into voluntary liquidation."

"We won't lose the house, will we?" I grabbed his arm.

He shook his head. "But there is a problem: if we go down this route it will cost us £5000."

"What? How can we get that sort of money if we are broke?" I asked in despair.

"Well, if I am going to live in Switzerland I won't need my car, so that should pay towards it plus I have some tax and VAT I have to pay." I squeezed Joseph's hand, as I knew how much the car meant to him. I felt ill with worry, but knew that to get through this we had to be positive and now wasn't a time to mope. Joseph decided to go to Switzerland for a week and to register with the selective agencies that may potentially find him work.

CHAPTER SIXTEEN – THE COFFEE JAR

Joseph advertised his car, a Honda sports type, at a bargain price of £6000, as we needed a rapid guaranteed sale. We placed it in a car trader magazine together on the Friday and just hoped it would sell. It was Saturday night and we were watching *Britain's Got Talent* when the silence in the lounge was suddenly shattered. I looked around. Joseph sat with his head in his hands weeping his heart out. I immediately put my arm around him. "I'm a failure. I don't want to sell my car, but I have to. It's more important I look after my family. I have failed. The kids aren't going to be proud of their dad. I don't want to go to Switzerland, and I shall miss you all." He rocked himself forward and Jo Jo ran and put her arms around him.

"We love you, Dad, and we are proud of you." She held him in her arms and I gulped as my husband looked so vulnerable whilst his little girl held him. I felt proud of her, and Tee Jay who looked really concerned had also come up and put his arm around him. I squeezed his hand and said, "Look, all of this doesn't matter. It is a house, that's all. If we have to go and live in a caravan, we will. You don't have to go."

"I've fought hard for this. We are not going to lose our home. I will go to Switzerland. I will miss you so much." He set off crying again and I squeezed his hand whilst at the same time tried to give Jo Jo and Tee Jay a reassuring squeeze on their arms. I knew I would have to talk to them the next day to reassure them that everything would be OK.

The following days were awful. We continued in our routine, but all the time we were all clock-watching and dreading the day he was going. It was good news on Tuesday, as we received a telephone call that someone was interested in his car. They arranged to come on the Tuesday night to pick it up. Joseph was upset but so relieved that we were going to get the money, as we needed £5000 to pay off the receivership fee. His relief turned to worry as the man didn't turn up and wouldn't answer his phone either. It was to be the Wednesday when he rang again and apologised, saying that he couldn't get the cash because his wife had gone into labour and could he come on Thursday with a banker's cheque. Joseph asked my advice. "Well, if it is a banker's cheque drawn on a bank, there should be no problem," I said. It was agreed that the car would be picked up on Thursday, and the only disadvantage for us was because it was Easter bank holiday the earliest we could bank the cheque was the following Tuesday, but at least we knew we had the £6000.

It was on Thursday that the chap turned up. Joseph had paid to have the car valeted, wanting to make sure it looked perfect for the buyer. I decided to keep out of the way and sat in my study when Joseph came through. "Is this alright?" he asked. He held out the banker's cheque. I examined it carefully, checking that it was drawn on the bank and that the sort code and account looked fine. It was drawn on Nationwide, and the payee was typed and professional. "Fine," I said, handing him the cheque. I turned to my computer and was interrupted again. "Can you come and help?" I walked into the kitchen to find the buyer sitting at our kitchen table filling in the appropriate forms. Joseph again asked me if everything was OK and I nodded. I followed them both out onto the drive, and the chap jumped into the car. Just as he was going to go I shouted to Joseph, "You did take your CDs out?" He put his hand to his mouth and knocked on the passenger window. "Sorry, I forgot to take my CDs." The man laughed as he gathered the CD collection, making sure he took the one out of the player. The chap waved and drove off quickly. "Isn't there anyone else?" I asked as we were in a remote spot. "No, they dropped him off," Joseph replied. We walked into the house together, feeling sad that we had lost our car, but happy we had the money.

The bank holiday passed and Joseph went to the bank to pay the money in. He wanted to sort the payment out before he left for Switzerland at the weekend. I started to do some ironing and sorting his clothes out for travelling. It was just after 11am when he arrived home and he came rushing to me. "I knew there was something wrong. I could feel it," he stated.

"What do you mean?" I asked.

"The cheque. It's not real."

"Don't be daft. It's drawn on the bank."

"The bank manager thinks it's a fraud."

"Well, where is it now?"

"They kept it. They are ringing their head office and will know by the end of the day," Joseph said.

"End of day, that's no good. You need to inform the police and the insurance company as soon as possible." I was shocked but knew that the sooner the police knew the more chance we had, if any, of getting the car back.

Joseph rang the bank back and they promised they would let him know as soon as possible. It turned into hours and when he rang again they eventually confirmed it was a fraud cheque. They insisted that an extremely professional gang must have been involved, as the cheque was flawless. The only giveaway was that the particular bank it was drawn on did not issue cheques. Joseph rushed to the local police station and also informed his insurance. I felt sick. I had witnessed him break down and cry because he had to sell his car, and now we had been victims of a fraud. We were fortunate because we had legal cover in the car insurance that the insurance brokers eventually decided they would pay up. But the drawback was that it was going to take time. The remaining days flew by and soon it was Saturday morning. Joseph had booked a one-way ticket to Switzerland and was determined he was not returning home until he had found a job. I hugged him, and as a last thought asked him how much money he was taking with him. He shrugged and turned out his pockets. He had less then £10. "You can't survive on that," I said.

"I am stopping with my brother or parents. I have no more," he replied. I realised we were in deep trouble. I went into my office and handed a couple of hundred that I had drawn out hoping it would keep me and the kids going. I pressed it into his hands. "Take it," I whispered softly. He had tears in his eyes as he put it into his wallet and I turned away to gather my own inner strength. The children came through and hugged him, and then he and I clung to each other and kissed each other softly. "Take care. I love you," I whispered again.

"I love you too." He hugged me and then we all made our way to the car. We had decided to drop him at the airport but not to go in, as waiting would have been too hard. The car journey was in silence, and as we waved goodbye I held back my emotions as I concentrated on driving home. Even Cara could not lift my spirits, but I knew I had to be strong and the kids had basketball in the next half hour. This helped us all take our mind off the present events.

Joseph rang later that evening and told me that the police had contacted him to inform him that the car had been traced heading south on the Thursday night. I believed it would be long gone and concentrated on asking him if he had settled in. He spoke to both children and promised to ring the next day.

It was to be a few days later that I received a telephone call from the police in Essex. I spoke to a very nice police lady who liaised with me because Joseph was abroad. "We have traced your car." She must have heard me gasp. "Where?" I asked.

"You won't believe it but we have traced it to a cargo shipment in Hamburg waiting to be shipped out to Jamaica. It's a shame, because if we had been a day earlier we could have stopped the shipment, but it is now in a massive container full of other cars waiting to be shipped on." I waited, having a gut instinct that there was more. "We are in a position to recall the cargo back here to recover your car, but because the container is full of vehicles it would cost the shipping company a lot of money to do this. The solution, with your permission, is that the shipping owner is willing to buy your car from you and then he can resell it to the buyer waiting in Jamaica. Would you and your husband be happy with this?"

"Would it be the same amount as we had originally sold it for?" I asked.

She laughed. "Yes, and of course he will try for less but I shall tell him if it isn't the full amount then you refuse and we will call the container back."

I felt relieved. "Another thing: will you be involved until we get the money? I would hate to agree then he take weeks to pay." I was anxious and trying hard to make sure I had everything covered.

"Yes, we will stay involved until the money has been transferred to your bank account. If you are happy to give me the go-ahead, I will start the process. I will contact you later." I thanked her and sat back, feeling so relieved that we might receive the money quicker than expected. We hadn't planned for all of this to happen, but after Joseph had left I started to receive more telephone calls from which I did not run away. I answered because I preferred to know exactly where we stood. It was bad that Joseph hadn't paid many bills for months, and I was sick with worry because every day I didn't know which demands were going to fall through the letterbox and who I would have to deal with on the phone. The next day the police rang me and after some necessary procedures the money was transferred over to our account for the car. It was a relief, but I was hesitant to use this money for the receivership fee as I was still unsure how deep the debts were. My feelings were that if Joseph could access some money from his family, it might cushion us until we could see the light and start to repay the money. I couldn't ask my own mum, as she had helped my sisters and I in the past, and Joseph's family was the last resort. We were fortunate that his mum lent him some money allowing him to pay the receivership fees and I managed to pay off some more of the personal debts. The company went into liquidation, and I felt guilty for the suppliers that were owed money, but at the same time relieved that he had managed to pay a lot of the debts off.

My emotions felt like they were in a tumble drier, rotating, twirling and then reversing one way and the other. I felt really angry with Joseph for allowing our financial situation to get so bad, yet then I accepted that we were in the middle of a double-dip recession and in fact many other people were experiencing similar difficulties. Then I would twirl and think of all the lying and deceit, and wondered if I could ever trust him again. When Martin visited, he told me he could understand why Joseph kept quiet. "It's male pride," he explained. "He wouldn't want you to know. He was trying to protect you. I wouldn't want Joanie to know."

I missed Joseph and was miserable. We would ring each other several times a day and both Jo Jo and Tee Jay would run to pick the telephone up. Tee Jay took his role of man of the house so seriously, and each night he would lock all the doors and take the keys out. He also refused to go to bed until he knew I was retiring. He took charge of putting the bins out and tried to do as many jobs as possible. I cleaned the house twice as much as I would have done, as in my mind I wanted to prove that we could keep everything perfect even without Joseph there. I coped well and had the support of Dr Lynn and Dr Dhanji. Maggie my diabetic nurse was sympathetic and I thought I was doing fine.

"Mum, can we have these?" Jo Jo asked. She was pointing to some yoghurts and I nodded to her. I looked across the frozen food aisle and spotted Tee Jay crossing items off the list. I felt proud of my children, as they had stepped up and each become more responsible. I walked up to the beverage shelf and was just about to place Joseph's favourite coffee into the trolley when I realised it would not be needed. The sight of a coffee jar suddenly brought many emotions to the surface and I looked away from the kids to gather myself, realising that it could be many months before we were together again. Simple routines like watching the kids play basketball had been smashed. My mind was all over the place. Would we only see each other for a few weeks in a year? When would he be home? I turned as Tee Jay pulled my arm. "Mum, do we need ketchup?" He made me smile; he loved ketchup with everything. "Yes, you'd better take some." We finished and went to pay.

Back at home I tried to place everything in perceptive. People did live apart: I thought of the Forces and how army wives managed, of people who went to work on oil rigs, people who worked on different shifts and hardly saw each other. We would get through this. I knew we would somehow.

CHAPTER SEVENTEEN – CONFIDENCE

It was challenging for me with Joseph away, as I disliked going to new places on my own and the kids still needed to be taxied to and fro to their various social outlets. We were lucky, as both children had made friends with some really nice people and they had already volunteered to help out with lifts. I was coping, but I had gone into an automatic mode and knew I was withdrawing back into my shell.

From publishing *A Fine Line* I had received thousands of messages and many people perceived that I had been brave and inspiring and had a lot of strength to fight through the difficult experiences. In my view my past had been the easy time, and even now I still argue with my consultant Dr Lynn that it was no big deal. In my eyes the difficult time was not experiencing the past, as I hadn't realised what was going on. I had suppressed most of it, was in denial and was on autopilot. The true battle to me was this part: the survival, and what helped me most was my children and family. I still lacked confidence, and I acknowledged that now with Joseph away I was even more tested, and I found myself becoming slightly paranoid and very self–conscious. Even filling up the car at a petrol station was uncomfortable. I told myself off, for I was in my fifties now, and had always filled my own car up. Yet in the last couple of years Joseph had volunteered to do it for me and now with him away I analysed who was at the pumps, who was going by and even surveyed the people who were passengers in the cars. I hated queueing to pay, as it meant someone could walk up behind me, so I tried to time it so that there was no one there. I didn't like to go to any new place as it was against my routine and challenged my confidence. Tee Jay was good, as he volunteered wherever possible to go into shops or pay at the till. He was very sociable and liked to chat to people. In return I found myself staying in the house more and even conscious of when I walked onto my driveway in case anyone passed on our lane or the neighbours were watching. The internet didn't help, as although I made some fantastic friends through sites such as Facebook, I found myself compensating for the deficit in my real social life by interacting more through social media. We were still in a vulnerable position with Joseph was still seeking work; the financial situation was fragile and the children had trouble at school as the standards of teaching had dropped in certain areas and Jo Jo had been quite ill with breathing problems.

***

"Bridget, your reactions to all of this are not appropriate." Dr Lynn sounded concerned yet factual.

"What do you expect me to do? Crawl into a corner and hide, or burst into tears?" I battled back.

"You are using the same method of coping as you did in the past, and I am worried you may become overwhelmed." Dr Lynn stared at me.

"I am fine. It won't help me worrying about it or breaking down, will it? I have to get on with it and manage through." I shrugged my shoulders, as I was starting to feel rattled. I continued before he could speak. "Look, you may get into a mess and fall apart and lean on the shoulders of others, and, yes, it may be healthy and you may receive the support and feel better for it. But – and it is a big but – I don't have anyone else to turn to, so there is no point in me cracking up and feeling sorry for myself." I stared defiantly at him, waiting for the response.

"Denying it all and suppressing your feelings won't work. You know that." Dr Lynn looked at me.

"Crying my eyes out and breaking down will not help me either," I argued back. "Things will sort themselves out. I am just going through a rocky patch." He smiled at me and I smiled back, noting that his grey hair had receded back more. Despite this, through the eighteen years I had been seeing him, he still remained a distinguished and attractive man. His tall, lean frame leaned towards me.

He spoke out. "It is OK to cry, you know." I shook my head and already I felt my barriers going up and my body steeling itself ready for any attack. The weird thing was that the kinder he or anyone else was, the more my guard was needed. He had joked once that if I used the box of tissues that was usually placed on the desk then I would be a step closer to being well. "What will you do if you lose your house?" It was a question I had repeatedly asked myself in the last few weeks. My main concern was not only to keep a roof over our heads but the welfare of all our animals, which must have totalled a hundred or more.

"I don't know at the moment. We will have to tackle it if and when the problem arises." Again I tried my best to keep calm and collected, as it was no good panicking and worrying about a problem that may not happen. "My main job is to keep the routine going the kids happy and stable and to act positive. Joseph is the one who is upset; he cried his eyes out when he had to go and he is not happy over there."

"When is he coming back?" Dr Lynn asked, crossing his legs the other way. I shuffled in my chair before I answered. "I don't know, that's why it is so hard, I don't know if it is weeks, months. I just don't know." I again was aware that I had steeled myself and was in the train of thought that if I had cut I would not have felt anything. I sighed and looked up to Dr Lynn. "OK, I'll admit it, I have been struggling the last week or so. At times I have wanted to go back to the woods and quarry. I have to fight those feelings off. I have felt the dark intensity and have wanted to run off, but again I don't want to as I love my kids and they're feelings and thoughts I don't want to have. I will fight them off. My diabetes and sugar count is all over the place: one day I need twice the insulin and the next I nearly don't need it. I know why I am like this, but I will manage it." I leaned back, relieved that I had spoken out.

Dr Lynn just looked at me and stayed silent. I sat and stared at the sign saying 'hot water' above the tap. "That's me. That's what I am in," I said. Dr Lynn looked puzzled. I explained and he looked to where I was staring. "Hot water, that's what I am in." I said it quietly.

He responded quietly. "It's like a repeat of your past, the way you are coping."

Again I shrugged my shoulders. "I am trying my best. That's all I can do."

"I'm just concerned it may overwhelm you." He looked intently towards me.

"I won't let it, I'm OK." I looked away, trying to gather my thoughts to stay calm and rational. I knew inside me I wanted to scream out. I didn't know whether we would lose our home; I didn't know if and when I would see Joseph again. I had over a hundred animals relying on my care and two children who needed stability after the time I had spent in hospital.

Dr Lynn spoke quietly and calmly. "Two weeks, ten o'clock." He patted me on my shoulder as he walked past me to the door. I grabbed my handbag and followed him through.

***

The gravel crunched as I pulled up on the drive. I never liked returning to an empty house, and I was glad when Asti and Cara barked to be let out of their cage. I let them out into the garden and stuck the kettle on. Always after I had seen Dr Lynn my mind was active as I was reflecting on our conversation and also trying to come to terms with the present situation. I took my cuppa into my study to read my emails, and just as I was replying to one the telephone rang. I answered it eagerly and Joseph spoke to me. "How are you?"

"Fine. Any luck?" I asked.

"No, I am going into Geneva later on today and will chase the agency." He spoke confidently.

"Aren't there others you can go to?" I asked.

"No, this is the main one, and I am sure they will have something in a week or so."

I sighed, as the waiting was stressful and I was impatient. I wanted him to be doing so much more.

"I go back to Mum and Dad's for a week then," Joseph said.

"Well, that won't help, will it?" I replied doubtfully, as I couldn't see how staying with his parents who hadn't got any internet or phone was going to be any good.

The weeks flew by and still Joseph had no interviews or work. I missed him dreadfully and I knew the children did too, as they would rush to answer the telephone. In some ways it was ironic because we had been going through a bad patch arguing and shouting, and Joseph had really taken it out on the kids. He would come in and shout for no reason. Tee Jay suffered the most, as he was always in the wrong. Even if he carried a dinner plate out, he would get told off for not holding it correctly. He would be told off for not clearing up quick enough, for placing the dishes in the wrong order in the dishwasher and silly little things that normally wouldn't have been picked up on. As mothers do, I was always trying to defend him and life had been very stressful. Now it was as if the kids and I had breathing space; we could relax and not jump when Joseph came into the room. It wouldn't matter if a cushion was out of place, or if the dog's paw went off the blanket. We could relax and I think we needed the breathing space. Life had become pretty unbearable, and I had tried to rationalise, thinking it was because of the financial difficulties. I was still dismayed at the deceit and the lies. It was also difficult trying to protect the children. I remembered at home when my dad had lost his job, my parents had tried to keep it quiet, yet as a kid you knew something was wrong. I remembered my dad sitting by the phone day in and day out. I thought about Jo Jo and Tee Jay a lot, and I thought it fair to them to be open about the situation but to also try to keep the pressure from reaching them. In some ways being open was better, as they could understand why we had arguments and why their dad was so stressed. I hoped it would help them realise that in no way they were to blame for any of the situation. Joseph and I had started to argue nonstop, and I had seriously thought about splitting up. Neither of us seemed happy, and I did not want to continue like we were, yet part of me held back because of the children and because although I disliked many of his actions I still loved him.

Now he was in Switzerland, and not knowing when we were going to see him next pulled us together. I kept really busy cleaning the house, running around after the children and still had the unpleasant business of not knowing who was going to ring or what demands were going to pop through the door next. Although Joseph had cleared most of the debts and everything was legal, I still felt very guilty because his business had gone into liquidation. I also felt threatened by the bank for the mortgage and had started to use the children's savings to keep the roof above our heads. I kept telling myself he would find work and it was a matter of waiting. I was dusting the lounge when the telephone rang, and I could see it was Joseph. "Hi," I breathed deeply as I was out of breath rushing for the phone.

"Hi, are you OK?"

"Yes, I was cleaning. I'm fine."

"The chap from the London agency has rung: they have an interview for me to possibly work in London in a wine shop." He hesitated, waiting for my reaction.

I took a deep breath. "I suppose any work is better than none at the moment, but it depends how much it is and travelling costs and residential cost."

"I know, and it also depends whether there is a chance to move up the ladder," Joseph replied.

"I think you ought to take the interview and then see what the prospects are and weigh it up."

"It will mean coming back and can we afford to travel backwards and forwards?" Joseph asked me.

"Well, if I was you, I would make sure you have visited all the agencies over there and chased up any opportunity possible, leaving your name in the right places if any work comes up in Switzerland and then come home. I would then go to London, weigh this job up, and then take it from there."

"I think you're right." Joseph's voice had brightened up enormously. "I'll telephone you later. Love you."

"Love you too." I placed the phone down and started dusting again. My steps felt lighter and in my heart I knew I was glad he was coming home. I was still worried, though, as I didn't think the London job would cover the debts.

I ran upstairs to tidy the bathroom, and as I cleaned the sink I caught sight of myself in the mirror. My long dark hair looked straggled on my shoulders and instead of nice tidy ends it looked like rats' tails. Most women loved going to the hairdresser; I hated it. I felt trapped. It was a place full of danger: there were scissors and sharps all over the place. I would look round and the glittering silver that lay dancing in their fingers or quietly placed on a work top would challenge my emotions. I would sense their presence close up, shoulder's length away, hovering and then as I heard the snip of the scissors and saw the dark hair fall I would be on a timer. During that time I knew I had to behave. I had to sit there and control the urge to run, the urge to grab the scissors. I attempted to block the images of blood trickling down my arms. "Where are you going on holiday this year?" I would look up at the hairdresser's idle chit–chat. "What are you going to do tonight? Going anywhere nice?" I would smile and answer politely back. All the time I was watching her moves, watching who was close by. I knew who was in the place and which hairdresser was using which utensils. As soon as the mirror was held up behind my head I was nodding smiling politely and ready to go.

It became easier when Jo Jo decided to have her hair done after me, as I would look across at her and smile. She unwittingly helped me ground myself and take my mind off the surroundings. When it was her turn I could breathe more easily and watch whilst they worked on her hair. I never felt threatened whilst watching my daughter, and I found it interesting watching how she interacted with the hairdresser, treasuring her little smiles and confident instructions.

***

I remembered several years back.

Flashback:
The nursing staff never lacked confidence. I had rung the ward as I was instructed to do when I felt bad, as I was on fast-track – a quick admittance to the ward if needed. It wasn't easy, as I had felt guilty at having to ring and never knew who would answer. "No, you don't want to come back in here. We haven't any rooms free, and if you do come back you will be in the men's side." I had received such a cold response from her, the nurse who had called me an opportunist and always called me trouble. I put the phone down, feeling heavy and even more desperate. I walked slowly into the kitchen, where I knew there was a piece of broken mug, and I used it across my arm. As the pressure caused my skin to split and cut, and after the cut released the blood, I started to feel lighter. The intensity disappeared and I quickly pulled my sleeve down and put the kettle on to make a drink. I sipped my tea slowly and watched the television. It didn't work. I was too agitated to sit and watch anything, thoughts of going into the woods engulfed me and the quarry intruded into my mind. I paced up and down and wondered whether to ring Joseph. I knew he was busy at his shop, the kids were at primary school and I didn't want any of them to know how bad I was feeling. I went into the kitchen and called Amba to me. She came ambling up, wet nose straight into my hands, tail wagging. I knelt down beside her and she immediately cuddled up to me. I hugged her close, my hands ruffling through her fur. I reached out and stroked Asti, who had come up pushing at me too. Both dogs seemed to know when I needed their love. Petrus meowed and I half laughed. "I haven't forgotten you." I picked her up and cuddled her, and she purred and kissed me with her nose. I placed her onto the settee and I rushed into the kitchen to make sure the mug pieces had been thrown away and out of sight. I was still fighting the intense thoughts, and although the animals were helping I so wanted to go into the woods. The quarry pulled me every time I was feeling low. I couldn't rationalise this, and why it did. I had been to the woods several times with my parents when I was a kid. I

124

remembered my sisters and I running through the trees and hiding in the huge brackens of ferns. I also remembered going with Sandra and walking through with the dogs. I wondered if it was the huge trees and nature pulling me. Was it nature's way of telling me my time had come? I didn't like the thoughts, and I again tried to shrug them off. The next day I had to see Andrea and I knew I wasn't good as I went to sit in the room with her. She stared at me and I sat silently. I couldn't sit still, and kept rubbing my arms. Every time she went to speak, I jumped. I sat and stared and it was as if I was staring down at myself. My mind was in circles. I needed to get home to the kids, but I was scared, I was frightened, and I felt desperate. I wanted to talk to Andrea. I wanted to tell her that I needed help, then I thought of the nurse, the 'no room available' and the spiteful tone in her voice telling me I would be in the men's side. I questioned in my head whether I wanted to have someone like her in charge of me. I turned. Andrea was saying something and in that second I bolted for the door. Andrea got there first. "Bridget, we need to talk." She spoke softly and with her hand on my arm she led me back to my chair. I sat in silence listening to her. She was telling me I needed to be back in hospital. I wanted to argue, but I knew that she was right, yet at the same time I knew there was a danger there. It was nurses like her – the one who answered the phone – who took me to the edge. It was nurses like her who had made me want to cut. She stirred emotions in me that I hadn't felt before: a kind of hatred. It meant I wanted to cut. I wanted to see the red of the blood, and when I was trapped I needed to break out. Andrea and Dr Lynn were so nice, but they only visited for an hour at a time even if it was daily, and it was nurses like *her* who were in charge. I did end up back in hospital and I broke out, bolting down the stairs and jumping a flight at a time. I was incredibly fit for my age and could outrun most people. I managed to get out of the hospital gates and with many nurses chasing me I ran straight out into the road. I heard the screeching of brakes as my hands felt the bonnet hitting me. I fell to the floor. I was lucky the driver had braked in time and I half-crawled to the pavement and just sat there. I was trying to get my breath and held my head low. I heard a laugh and then Lee's voice. "Has she been hit?" He laughed as he asked. I felt like jumping up and spoiling his delight, but I kept my head low and allowed myself to be led away back to the ward.

***

CHAPTER EIGHTEEN – BACK HOME

We sat in the car watching people come and go as we waited for Joseph's train to arrive. "Can we go over there, Mum? " asked Jo Jo. I looked at my watch: there were still a few minutes to go and it was chilly. "Give it a couple of minutes," I replied. Tee Jay was already zipping his coat up and he opened the car door. "Mum said wait." Jo Jo leaned over and pulled the door to again. Both children sat silent and still. "Oh, come on then." I grabbed the keys and jumped out, and by the time I had shut the door they were already walking onto the platform, the train approaching in the distance. We stood back watching the doors slam as people clambered out. Faces watched from the train as people hugged each other and others just walked through during a daily routine. "There he is!" Tee Jay shouted, and he had already gone. I watched as Joseph put down his suitcases to hug his son. Jo Jo followed and after hugging her he picked the case up and walked towards me. Tee Jay took his case and he gave me a kiss and we hugged, clinging tightly, and for those few seconds in a world of our own. "Come on," I said and grabbing his hand led him over to the car. The kids were excited and already in the back seat. Joseph climbed into the passenger side and I turned the key to take my family home.

"Good luck, Daddy!" both kids shouted in unison as they left for school. Joseph had his interview in London and we were all rooting for him. Life had turned back to normal, and I rushed back from the school, as I had to take Joseph to the same station to catch the London train. He looked smart in a dark grey suit and new shoes. I wished him luck and returned home. Apprehension clung in the air. I went outside and started to clean the animals out, brushing hard and fast. I had taken the telephone outside and I clock-watched, knowing that he would be out of the interview at three. It was dead on three when the phone went and I picked it up anxiously. "How did it go?"

"Not sure. I managed to answer all their questions but they didn't seem that interested." His voice dropped and I took a deep breath.

"Well, you've done your best. You will just have to wait and see; we all will. I'll be at the station at seven o'clock. Love you."

"Love you too." He put the phone down.

I finished off the animal pens and fed the dogs and rushed inside to put the kettle on. I felt a bit down and very anxious. I realised that I had thought Joseph would get the job easily. The door banged and the kids came through to the kitchen, throwing their bags onto the table. They both rushed up to give me a kiss. "How did school go?" I asked. "Fine!" they both shouted in unison. I laughed as they both went running upstairs. "Change out of your school clothes!" I shouted after them. "OK!" they both shouted again, and I laughed as I went into the kitchen.

Joseph shrugged his shoulders as our eyes met, and I grabbed his arm. "Come on, tell me at home." He explained over dinner how the interview went. It didn't sound good and I tried to cheer him up.

"Look, to be honest, by the time you have taken away tax, the train fares and the accommodation, it still would not have been enough. It might have done you a favour." I stared at him. It was no good pretending things were going to turn out fine; we had to be realistic. The next few days we talked, we fell out and we talked. "You need to go out and talk to people. They might give you some ideas." I looked at Joseph seriously. "Be honest with yourself. You have tried all the agencies in England, you have been to Switzerland, and you have even placed your name for worldwide vacancies. Think about it: you even considered China and America. We haven't found anything. Everywhere seems to be struggling; we are in a recession and there are a lot of people looking for work. You need to chat to people and try to find some footing." Joseph looked at me and I could tell from his body language that he was fed up. He had started to go to bed in the afternoons, and although I sympathised with him, I was also getting annoyed, as I knew that wouldn't solve our problems. "I am going to go to see Geoff tonight," he said.

"Good, I'll keep the dinner in the oven for you." I kissed him on the cheek and turned to finish my jobs.

The idea worked, as when Joseph came in later he was nearly bouncing as he walked. "I've been talking to Geoff and Janine, and they both said I am wasted working for others and that with my expertise I should be working for myself, and to try to start up again. Geoff said he would support me and pass the word on." I smiled, as it was the first time in ages that he looked himself. I kept quiet and let him continue. " I have been thinking: I have a friend who I can contact who has a decent list of wines he may let me sell them with him." I nodded in agreement and was pleasantly surprised by his enthusiasm.

In the next few days we received a response that Joseph had failed to get the job in London. I believed it was meant to be, and was happy that Joseph was building his confidence back to sell wine again. I believed his expertise would have been underestimated elsewhere. He was one of the best wine experts in the world, and having worked in the top Michelin star restaurants such as La Gavroche, L'Orangerie in Hollywood, been a guest taster on *Masterchef* and worked on television as a wine expert for years and in other famous places, I wanted him to be appreciated for his expertise.

Joseph had some meetings with his friend, and within a couple of weeks had started to set up a new business. He was lucky that some of the pubs and businesses he had supplied before wanted to use his expertise again and started to use wines from his list. He also started to receive requests for his wine-tasting evenings and quietly and slowly he started to build the business and his confidence back up.

One of the drawbacks was that we only had one car between us, causing stress and inconvenience because our nearest bus stop was a couple of miles away. It meant that Joseph and I had to communicate well, as I had hospital and other medical appointments and the children had their social timetables and of course Joseph needed the car for his work. Although our home was in a beautiful setting, the biggest drawback was the lack of social contact. There were a few neighbours along the lane and years back we had some good social gatherings and partied through the night. Now no one had time for each other. A result of having only one car also threatened my confidence, as it was an easy excuse not to go out because Joseph needed it so much. I already had to push myself to even see my friends, and now on the rare occasion I felt up to going out I was lucky if the car was free. I turned more and more to the internet, where I had managed to make some really good friends. I worked on my blogs and my book page. Through my psychology degree and with searching for positive messages to post on my site, I started to learn more about myself and to some extent I could justify some of my past actions. It was also through messages I received from people that I started to learn I was not alone. The biggest problem was the stigma mental health had, and I remembered back to when an agency nurse had to look after me.

*****

Flashback:
She stood by the door and I could tell from her body language that she was not at ease, her fingers touching the tag. She kept looking out down the corridor and I could also tell she was scared.
"Do you want us to go and make a cup of tea?" I asked. Her eyes widened as if I had suggested the impossible. She nodded and she waited for me to walk past her and followed me closely at arm's length to the kitchen. There

were no other patients in there and I selected two clean mugs. "Tea or coffee?" I looked at her.

"Coffee, two sugars, thanks," she spoke hesitantly. I threw a teabag in one mug and a good spoonful of coffee in another. "Hey, tea, please!". I looked across as Melanie, another nurse, was shouting across to me. I raised a thumb up and selected another mug and made an extra tea. On the way back I crossed the reception to the nurses' room and passed her the mug. "Thanks, Bridget." She smiled at me. "You're welcome," I replied as I walked back to my room. I sat on the bed and offered my level-one companion a biscuit. She was again hesitant, but then took one and smiled. She came into the room and sat on the chair between my bed and the door. I grinned and sat leaning back on my bed, dunking my biscuit into my tea. "You looked shocked," I said to her. There was a silence and she drank her coffee. She laughed awkwardly and I waited. "I didn't know what to expect. It's not how I thought," she replied.

"OK, I won't take offence, but what did you expect?" I laughed as I talked to her. She didn't respond.

"I bet you expected me to be banging my head against the wall, or talking to myself or trying to run up the walls, rolling eyes. What else can I say?" I looked at her, my eyebrows raised.

"I did expect you to be like that." She frowned as she talked. "I was scared but I didn't want to show it."

I offered her another biscuit. "Well, sorry to disappoint," I said.

She laughed and took another biscuit from the packet. "I'm sorry. I feel an idiot, but that's how I had pictured it." She jumped as there was a massive yell from one of the patients and a tag was pulled, alarms sounding with lots of banging and shouting.

"If I was you I would ignore it and stay here. You're not supposed to leave me, and they will block off the area anyway," I told her. I was right and a nurse came down to tell us not to leave the room. After being in and out of the psychiatric unit for the last few years, I knew that the patient who had tried to escape would be sedated and placed in seclusion. It was not nice to see anyone being forcefully injected and it actually traumatised me the times I had witnessed it. Some nurses were very professional and made sure it was private and calmed the patient down, while others just wound them up more and purposely humiliated them, injecting them with no privacy and exaggerating their power as they injected. At times like this I had felt physically sick and when a disruption happened I preferred to stay in the privacy of my room. My nurse looked nervous. "It's OK. It will all be over in a short time," I told her.

"The nurses told me I had to be really careful with you," my agency nurse said. "They said you were really nice, which made it harder as I could easily be off my guard." She looked at me questioningly.

"They are right. I can bolt and I can act out, but I am not doing any of my therapy work I went out earlier on so I don't feel trapped and as long as nothing kicks off really bad, I don't feel too bad. If I am bad I usually get agitated and can start to shake. So long as you stay that side of me I should be fine. I know it sounds bad but I had an agency nurse the other week who was supposed to be watching me and whilst we went out to reception, she left me to go and look out of the window. I know I shouldn't have, but in that split second the door was there and I was unguarded so I walked quietly out and then bolted up the corridor and escaped. Although that time I got into massive trouble."

"Why?" she asked me.

"Because I hadn't planned it. I acted on impulse and I fled, and when that happens the adrenalin rush kicks in. To be honest it's like being dissociated – you aren't thinking straight, as it was on an impulse, and I walked around not knowing why or where I was going. It was later on that I rang the ward and I was in real trouble. Even the nicest of nurses were so angry with me." I paused as I still felt it had been an injustice.

"Why?" My agency nurse, who was quite petite and very pretty, stared at me with wide open eyes. She brushed her dark hair away as she waited for me to answer. I frowned as I remembered the reaction of the nurses. "Apparently this agency nurse told them I had pushed her over and then I had run. She burst into tears and told them I had hurt her. She received the sympathy vote and of course I was the bad person. When I came back they didn't believe my version, although I even told them to ask one of the patients who was sitting by and saw it all." I threw my hands into the air. "Think about it: if I had pushed her over, she would have pulled her tag or shouted out. It would have made a commotion and I would never have got out. Also I can't even stand on an ant. I dislike hurting anything or anyone, and I wouldn't push someone on purpose. It isn't in me to do that." I paused and then continued. "She wasn't doing her job right. She shouldn't have left me and of course she would have been in trouble. It was easier for her to lie. I didn't do it on purpose. I wouldn't plan it like that. I would not want anyone to get into trouble; I acted impulsively." The agency nurse shrugged her shoulders and put her mug onto the side. "The worst thing was that one of the nurses who was always nasty to me made a right big song-and-dance about it. She came in to complain to my consultant when I was talking to him. She called me an opportunist and, yes, she was right in a way, as it was an opportunity and I took it. But I didn't plan it. Some of the nurses here think just because we have mental health problems that we are trouble. They think we cause trouble on purpose. She calls me a troublemaker. They also think we haven't a brain. She is always ordering people about as if they were at school." I laughed as I was contemplating which was the worst nurse. "There is Sheila as well. She will talk to you like you are about five years old and will hold your hand to walk you anywhere. Actually when you are feeling low it is nice to have the contact, but when you are OK, it is very patronising and humiliating. Also most of the nurses will let you go to the loo on your own so long as you leave the door open a little, but Sheila, she comes right in and stands right near you. I know." I laughed at her face. "You might have to do that. I am OK as at this time I am allowed to shut the door. They have put me on a trust and I try my hardest not to break it. But then there are the power trips of the nurses who like to order you to keep the door wide open even when there are other patients walking by. I try to time my needs to who is with me and who is next. I ask who is going to level-one me, and I set a timetable for myself." My nurse laughed and for the first time she looked relaxed. "I wonder what your timetable was for me?" I laughed this time and we were both laughing when there was a knock at the door. "I timed a cuppa, as I didn't know you!" I shouted after her as my next level one came on duty.

***

I felt a bit depressed. There was a lot going on, and I had also had some recent bad reviews for my book. My consultant and even people who I didn't really know from my book page had told me to ignore the reviews. I was told that there would be people who had issues with their own life and who wouldn't like to see someone doing well. There would be people who would dislike the writing and there would be some people who took delight in being nasty. I was warned to ignore the worst, but it was hard when my book was true and so personal. The book did receive an amazing positive response and this motivated me and helped me to deal with my past a little more. Yet despite the warnings to ignore the bad reviews they knocked me down and I took them to heart. It was months later when I had received thousands of messages that were positive and helpful, and from people that were thanking me for helping them, that I managed to place things into perspective. I told myself that if my book had helped one person then it was worth it, and the bonus was it turned out that it had helped many more people. Again, through these messages I also learned that it was reassuring when somebody else had felt similar emotions. It seemed to justify my reactions and emotions. I personally disliked labelling and generalising, yet when someone else could relate to my experiences it was a relief. I learned through so many people that feeling rejected at the slightest signal was common. So many others who had suffered from abuse looked for reasons for others to reject them. I started to understand myself a little more. It took a long time, but I started to learn that not everyone was out to use me or hurt me. I started to be more open and learned that I had to give myself more credit – that I was worth a lot more, and when I saw a signal that in the past I would have immediately taken as a rejection, I started to look for other reasons for that signal. Other feelings started to make sense as well: I realised that many people still felt guilty at allowing the abuse to happen, and when I read their accounts I was horrified that they should feel guilty. It was clear that they had been groomed to such an extent they didn't realise it was happening. They were powerless. It was easy to understand and see why it had happened, and in many cases it was so sad as the people who could have helped again looked away. It was through repeated accounts and experiences that the pieces started to fit together. I could see how denial and suppression were the enemies, and I could see what caused these enemies to battle on as they were coping mechanisms. Through many of the messages I could sense an urgency that the person wanted to be well, that they wanted to get better but their self esteem had been knocked to such a low that they were vulnerable. Even though they could take so many steps forward, it only needed a slight knock for them to fall to the bottom again. A situation that caused me to fall backwards and caused so much damage and mistrust was ironic, because where it took place was in the building and environment that was supposed to be helping me get better.

CHAPTER NINETEEN – THE DECISION

I took a liking to the new patient and watched with interest as he was shown to his bed. Then it dawned on me he was shown to his bed in the ladies' dormitory. I knew I often had a room on the men's side because all the ones on the ladies' were taken up. Yet the nurses would not place a male in the ladies' dormitory. I obviously had it wrong. I soon had the chance to confirm my mistake, as he turned out to be a she: a young kid of about eighteen years old with the cheekiest grin I had ever seen. "Hi, I am Billy," she said, coming through the door into my room.

"Hi Billy. I am Bridget," I said with a smile.

"Can I sit down?" she asked.

I gestured with my arm to the chair, but already she had sat on my bed and was laughing at the level one nurse. "Why have you got one of them?" She rather rudely pointed at Irene, who was sitting at the door reading a magazine and keeping an eye on me.

"They like my company," I replied, winking at Irene, who started laughing. Billy also laughed and shrugged her shoulders.

"Will you come and play football with me and a couple of nurses later on? They said we could." She turned to me. "They said we could go early afternoon after the lunch breaks and before the shift gets changed." I nodded as it sounded like fun. I just hoped that Dr Lynn or Andrea wouldn't come in that time. I was reassured by Mel that they would call me if this happened, and so there I was playing football and really enjoying it. Two of the nurses had joined in and Billy was really a good player. We also had a couple of the other patients who had come for a game and we played for a good hour. We then went

133

back upstairs to the ward. Billy went to her dormitory and I returned to my room and switched the television on. It had only been a few minutes before Billy appeared with her Xbox. "Can I play it in here?"

"Yes, course you can." I was pleased, needing any extra entertainment to relieve the boredom. Billy sat on my bed and played several games. I watched, bemused and glad of her company. She hadn't been there long before Dr Lynn appeared. He walked through and already Irene was beckoning to Billy to leave the room. "Who is that?" Dr Lynn asked me.

I laughed. "Oh, that's Billy. She is fairly new here."

Dr Lynn frowned. "I've told you before. Try to keep yourself to yourself. A word of advice: keep your distance."

I frowned back. "Why? She wasn't doing any harm."

"I've warned you." He sat back and started to ask me about the lifeline and some of the drawings on the bed. Andrea appeared, and she smiled and pulled up a chair. They both chatted and talked to me about my therapy and where we were with it, and after Dr Lynn had left I turned to Andrea. "Why doesn't he want me to mix with the other patients?" I asked.

"I think he was just looking out for you and wants you to concentrate on your therapy. Patients are going to distract you from your work, and come on, Bridge, you know you are vulnerable." She smiled and I knew deep down they were just looking out for me. After she had gone I went with Irene, who had drawn the short straw of looking after me most of the day, to the kitchen to get a drink.

"They told me to stay away from Billy," I said to her, wanting to know what her response would be. She passed me a mug of tea and walked back with me to my room.

"Well, they know best," she replied.

"Yes, but Billy is OK and I get bored. It's nice to have her around."

"Well, just be careful," Irene replied.

I continued to let Billy use my TV for her Xbox, and we talked quite a bit. It was unfortunate that she had just jumped on the bed beside me and started to talk when Dr Lynn walked in. He stopped and looked and she jumped off the bed, leaving her games, and went up the corridor. He looked sternly at me and I sat feeling embarrassed yet quite defiant. "I can't see the harm. She keeps me company and you told me I have to start trusting people." I was already making excuses.

"Talk to the nurses; talk to Andrea. Have your friends in, but just be careful. Remember patients are in here for a reason and many are quite ill." He had sat down and I nodded and sat quietly.

Later that afternoon Billy came in. I glanced at her. I could see why I'd thought she was a boy, as she dressed in army clothing, had short hair and her clothes camouflaged any feminine characteristics. "What's up?" she asked.

"I've been warned not to see you as much," I replied.

"Well, fuck that for a start," she said.

"It's because they want me to concentrate on my work, and not get diverted," I replied. I wasn't going to say anything else.

"Well, you don't have to work all the time, do you?" she replied. "Fuck him, thinks he is better than anyone else."

"He has helped me a lot," I replied defensively. She shrugged her shoulders and walked out of the room.

She soon came back. "Come here."

"Why?" I asked.

"You'll see." She grabbed my hand and literally pulled me off the bed and walked me along the corridor, and with Irene following, pulled me right across the reception area.

"What?" I didn't get chance to finish my sentence, as I suddenly saw what she had done. I had gone with her, still holding hands, as I thought she was leading me to something on purpose, and all the time she knew Dr Lynn was still in the nurses' staff room. He looked up to see me holding hands with her, standing in the reception area. "Come on," said Billy defiantly, and she pulled me towards the kitchen. I walked through and laughed, but deep down I was feeling guilty as I thought Dr Lynn deserved more respect than that. Irene raised her eyebrows at me and I concentrated on making a drink.

All afternoon, I worked hard on my therapy and drew and attempted to write about parts of my past. By evening time I was tired and decided to retire to bed early. By coincidence Irene was back on night shifts having done the early shift that day. She sat outside my door as my level one, reading a magazine. I liked Irene. She must have been in her sixties, with white hair and a lovely smile, and she was one of the kindest nurses on the ward. She shared her tea bags when the ward had run low and laughed and joked with me at times. My light was switched to low and I pondered whether I wanted to go to sleep or watch some more television.

Suddenly Billy pushed through and sat on my bed. "Do me a favour. Read this. I haven't trusted anyone else."

She gave me a notebook and I looked at the scribble on the front. "Are you sure? It looks personal."

"Please. I want to share it with you, then you will know why I am here."

I took the notebook from her, propping myself up a little on my pillow and started to read. It was hard reading what she had suffered. Unexpectedly, she lay down and put her head on my pillow. I went to react and it was too late.

* * *

Her warm smoky breath filled the air. I could feel her hands coming down under the sheets and I gripped hard onto the notebook. At the same time I could feel her fingers reaching out to me. She was touching me inappropriately and already my body had frozen. I heard, "She shouldn't be in there", and saw Zena walk by on the quarter of an hour routine check. She was telling Irene off. I wanted it to stop, she reminded me of Sandra. Yet this all seemed to be happening in the distance. I was calling out and screaming but it was in my head. My body felt trapped and I couldn't move. I was willing Irene to turn and shout "stop!", but she was too busy reading. I couldn't turn to face Billy. I knew her head was touching mine, and her hands were touching me under the covers. The smoke confused me, as I turned to look I could see Sandra and I was once again in a very dark place. I was sweating and as I looked up to the ceiling it was as if my body had parted from my soul. Time passed me by and it could have been five minutes or five hours; I had no idea. All of a sudden she was gone.

* * *

I lay back, exhausted, and eventually I fell asleep. The next few days were confusing, as I didn't want to believe that this could be happening to me again. I bottled it up and I felt sick. All I could think about was that smell. Anywhere I went I could still smell that breath of smoke. I could feel the shock of that head on my pillow and that smell of smoke. Sandra danced in and out of my mind. The image of Billy's face on the pillow haunted me and I could feel the events underneath the sheets. My feelings turned to distress and I tried to talk it over with the nurses.

Their reaction was unexpected, and they just told me they would talk to Billy. Even when I spoke to Andrea her reaction was, if it did happen then I deserved it. My feelings turned towards hate to Billy, but then also horror as I remembered reading what she had suffered. I then felt protective towards her as my mind tried to justify her actions. She was just a kid. She had been

136

through hell. She smiled at me and even told me the nurses had been to ask her what happened that night. "I told them," she said, and smiled. I felt sick and had to turn away. It was later that week that Dr Lynn had allowed me to go home for the weekend. I was unsettled even at home. Talking to Jo Jo and getting Tee Jay ready for nursery, I could still smell that smoke.

Once the kids were at nursery I set about tidying the house. I couldn't settle. Joseph had gone to work and I was left alone. The smell haunted me and even outside the pungent bitter smell of the tobacco was as clear as if someone was holding a cigarette under my nose. I could feel...

I walked up to the first lake. It was quiet and there was nobody around. The middle looked deep and as the waves rippled around the edges, I knew I wanted to stop the smell. I wanted to stop the feeling. I wanted to die. I couldn't understand why Irene hadn't stopped her. Why Zena, who had told Irene off, had still continued to walk by. Why the nurses didn't want to know. I questioned it and I felt her hands. I smelt the smoke and I thought about me. I realised that in all the time they were trying to get me better it was because it was a job: they were paid to look after me. The fact that people had hurt and abused me had given them work. But now it was a patient in their care who had abused me. Now it was a patient who had been allowed to jump in my bed even though I was on level one. She'd been allowed to get under the sheets and...

I realised to my sadness that they didn't care about this event. To them, this event was best forgotten, denied, and it hadn't happened. Where did that leave me? Nowhere. People didn't really care, and I was going to be thrown aside for the sake of someone's reputation and job. I didn't blame Dr Lynn, as he hadn't been there. I liked Irene so much and wished she had stopped it, but she was being kind in letting Billy come in, and Billy had just wanted to be close and looked after. I thought of Sandra. She had been close. The smoke again reached into my lungs and I needed to get rid of it. I started to walk into the water and the depth and cold made me jump. I slipped and went right under, and as I floundered to get a grip, I thought of Jo Jo and Tee Jay and realised what I was doing was wrong. In that split second I realised that I didn't want to die. I wanted to live, but I didn't want the black. The black flooded my mind more than the water in my lungs. I so wanted it to go. I pulled myself up and wearily and suddenly walked back along the hidden track to my home. Once in the corridor I

137

stripped my clothes off and placed them in a washing machine, eager to hide my weakness. I showered and dressed. I rang Dr Lynn. He was my safety net and my lifeline, and I knew he would understand that I was suffering and help me get through. However, his response was not the usual. He was rushing.

"Look, Bridge, we will talk about this on Monday." He had put the phone down, and once again the despair pulled at me. I wanted to cut to take away the pain. I rang the helpline I had been given for a lady in hospital who I had been told could help inpatients with legal advice. I was given an appointment for the following week.

***

I ended up being recommended a solicitor who decided he would take up my case. I thought of all the sayings and morals like, 'Do not bite the hand that feeds you'. I felt guilt, I felt unrest and I felt bitter. I did not want to take legal action against the people who had helped me so much, but I felt it wrong that I, as a vulnerable patient in hospital for therapy to come to terms with my awful history, had been cast aside because what had happened may threaten the ward. I was on level-one, which meant the closest of surveillance, and even after I had gone to bed, another patient had been allowed to come into my room and subject me to the same horrors of the past that I was having therapy for. It really hurt. Dr Lynn was shocked when he found out I was taking legal action, and tried to persuade me to drop the case. "You will not be able to go through

with it. You will become more ill. If you had come to me we could have talked it through. I could have taken it further." I had looked at him, and it had hurt because I knew I *had* gone to him, and he hadn't wanted to know. None of the medical staff had wanted to know, even my favourite nurses who I knew were decent human beings. It had thrown me and I had questioned myself. I had asked myself whether I had deserved it. I had been warned, but had I deserved to be…

I thought about it and decided that if it had been another patient I would have been horrified. I decided to continue with the case and the solicitor started to ask for all the medical background and information necessary. The months passed by, and as the solicitor worked on the case I ended up paying fees amounting to several thousand pounds. Friends around me were divided: some told me to give up because of the cost and others told me to continue. Deep down I knew that I had to fight for my principles and morals. It had been wrong, and should never have happened. My biggest regret was that the nurse who was in charge of the ward was one of the nicest nurses I had ever met, and I liked Irene so much. I wished Zena had taken more action. I wished, but I couldn't turn the clock back. I also decided that if I won the case it wasn't about the money. I would have had my costs back and given them any money back. It was about the principle.

I liaised with Dr Lynn all the way. He spoke to the solicitors and he also tried to protect me. I was in a peculiar situation. The case had come to a head. I had to make a choice either continue with the case, which had now come so far Dr Lynn would not have been able to continue to be my consultant, or drop the case. I had spent a lot of money and I had to weigh everything up. I talked it through with Paula, who had been with me all the way through, and I also talked it through with Joseph. I decided I needed Dr Lynn more than my pride, and although I was reluctant I also thought that I had made my point. I dropped the case.

***

Reflecting back on the case, I knew it left me feeling hurt, worthless and bitter at the time. Yet as time passed by I managed to see it in a different light. In my mind all it had needed was an apology from the staff to make me feel worthy, and a sign of regret that it happened. Yet the real cost of this to them would have been too much: an enquiry would have had to be held and there were so many consequences along the line. Also, even though Dr Lynn was not there at the time, potentially if he had stuck up for me and things had gone the wrong way, he might have helped me, albeit at the risk of losing the chance to help many other patients. I had the choice of being the victim and feeling pretty bad, or letting it go. I also questioned whether if I had listened to Dr Lynn in the first place it would still have happened, but still believe even if I had wanted another patient to jump into my bed which I didn't. It should never have been allowed to happen.

***

Our situation at home placed me under a lot of stress, and I was worried I might crack up, especially as stressful times seemed to allow memories of the bad times to form. Yet with Joseph being back home, I intended us to rebuild our family life back together again.

CHAPTER TWENTY – REBUILDING

With Joseph back at home, we started to get our lives back together again. It wasn't easy, as the demand for money was more than our income and we had to count every penny. We changed our lifestyle and we bought food according to what was on offer. We planned our journeys as economically as we could, and the kids continued to share their lifts. We explained to Tee Jay and Jo Jo that we wouldn't be going on holiday, and although they were disappointed they were good about it. We will still have fun, I told them, and I just hoped the weather would be good for the summer. I also explained that Cara was still a puppy and it would not have been easy to have leave her with anyone as she was so mischievous and needed strong supervision.

As my psychology degree was out of the way, I had much more time on my hands, and I was on the internet probably a bit too much. Yet with increased communication and especially with many more people who had gone through similar ordeals, I continued to gain insight and this also continued my journey to understand myself and to attempt to overcome some of the problems that I still had. I still saw Dr Lynn every other week, and we still explored avenue after avenue. I relied on my visits to Dr Dhanji in between, and I sometimes questioned my reactions to Dr Lynn with her. Dr Dhanji was always very professional and never gave an opinion one way or another over anything Dr Lynn had said. I never expected her to, but just airing an issue helped me gain some insight. I sometimes gave myself the answer in how I addressed the issue to Dr Dhanji. If I addressed it strongly, I knew deep down there was extra meaning to it. If it didn't surface, it hadn't been that important or I had already settled it. Dr Dhanji also helped me a lot with my physical ailments, and she was someone I could turn to that made me feel I was not alone with my problems. I had a great professional relationship with her and as I waited for her today, I chatted to Julie the receptionist about the children's school, as her children had been to the same one.

"Do you let yours take alcohol with them to parties?" I asked her. I was a little uncertain, as Jo Jo had started asking us to get her some alcohol when she went to a party.

"Well, you have to." ," Julie said, and she echoed my thoughts. "They will never learn if you shield them. You have to let them find out for themselves." I nodded in agreement and sat back satisfied at the answer. "Remember next time you make her a coffee call her Nicole." Julie laughed she knew I was referring to Dr Dhanji who I thought was the spitting image of Nicole the pop star who featured on X Factor. She was very pretty with long dark hair and a brilliant figure. It was nice to be able to joke with the staff even though the professional boundaries were still upheld. It helped my confidence and self esteem. I sat back and waited and it wasn't long before Dr Dhanji beckoned me in.

"And how are you?" she asked as she sat back in her chair.

"Fine," I answered, and we both laughed as I always said "Fine". I chatted to her about Jo Jo and her hospital appointments, and mentioned how I was having trouble with both the kids' schools again. The standard of teaching was causing great concern, and I knew that many parents had taken their children out of the school. She read a proposed letter that I had written to the school expressing my concerns, and we discussed how the potential consequences affect the children. She also advised me on my Menieres Disease, which had flared up again. I was sure it was due to the extra stress we were under. I left satisfied that I had crossed off another thing to do on my list and after calling in for my prescription I headed home.

I found it very difficult at home: on the one hand I was pleased Joseph was back, yet now he seemed to be everywhere I looked. 'Every step I take...' I thought.

In my head I was trying to be rational, give it time, but it was hard on all of us. I was impatient and as much as I knew and understood that Joseph had to build the business and he wouldn't always have work to do, I found it stressful. Joseph started to go to bed more and more in the afternoon and with increasing bill demands I felt under pressure. I started to do more and more work around the house and in the paddock, and basically ignored medical advice to take it easy. The work kept the demons away, and as I weeded the garden I tried not to notice the closed curtains above me. Joseph and I started to have many rows. The most stupid thing of all was that most of our arguments started from something really trivial. I believed part of our problem was misunderstanding through lack of communication. I also believed that every family had arguments, and when we tore each other apart we actually grew stronger together afterwards.

September arrived, and with it so did a new school term – Jo Jo's last school year. It was frightening how the time had flown by. Tee Jay had spent his fourteenth birthday party at home in his new tent. The cats and dogs slept in there and Tee Jay spent most of the summer nights camping out. Jo Jo decided she wouldn't bother with a sixteenth birthday party, worried about people getting drunk at home, and we just didn't get round to booking anywhere as there had been many problems with kids her age getting drunk and causing damage. We didn't want her to miss her sixteenth party, and Tee Jay and Molly, one of Joelle's best friends, arranged a secret party for her at the house after school. Jo Jo had no idea, and had decided to stay at school to attend a netball match, while about twenty of her friends all invaded the house. I had never laughed so much to see them all trying to hide in the lounge. We had a six-foot-plus lad called Sean on the sofa under the cushions. We had another lad hiding under the beanbags, girls behind the chairs, peeping from the curtains, and lads under the table. The suspense was fantastic. "Surprise!" we all shouted as the door opened and Jo Jo walked in. The look on her face told me we had done the right thing. She later told me it was the best party she had ever had. She had a barbecue and they all went for a dip in the pool, then all posed the Usain Bolt stance on the neighbouring walls. Joseph joined in, playing football, and when our greenhouse smashed it was the kids laughing at Joseph's football skills. It was a night to be remembered.

Both kids settled back into their new classes reasonably well, and as the nights started to draw in, I prompted them to think about what they would like for Christmas. "We haven't any money," replied Jo Jo. "So what's the point?" She was stating this as a fact and wasn't being awkward.

"The point is we haven't been on holiday, we have had a pretty tough time this year and the one day of the year I do want to enjoy is Christmas. Bear with me and have a think. We might not have much, but what I do want to get is something you need, not just a trivial gesture." I turned to look at Tee Jay, who was playing on his iPod. "What would you like?" I asked him. I should have known his answer, as it hadn't changed for the last few years. "An ostrich," he replied, grinning. I laughed and raised my eyebrows. "Come on, Mum, I could ride it," he added. Jo Jo stormed out of the room shaking her head; she could never understand her brother's passion for animals. "Think again," I replied to Tee Jay and smiled at him as I left the room.

I was just grateful we were all together and that Joseph was at home and not in a foreign country. This year was my turn to have my mum stay and I knew we would make the day special whatever we did.

The kids' basketball was in full swing again and like many other parents we were busy travelling to and from places as they competed at different levels and events. I loved to watch both my kids play, and I remembered Denny's words, which were: 'Make the most of it whilst you can. Before you know it they are grown up and gone.' I did try to make the most of it and was always amazed at how little the younger kids looked every time a new season started. I made friends with some of the parents whose children played in the same teams as Jo Jo and Tee Jay, and to my surprise when I accepted a lift to a local rugby match to watch Tee Jay play, my travelling companion turned out to be my old art teacher. It was a major shock, but a pleasant one. He hadn't changed that much, and I would have recognised him even though it was forty years on. I used to draw all the time when I was younger and in the hospital it was my main way of communicating.

***

The same way my first book was on auto-pilot, where the words tumbled out quicker than I could think, my drawings appeared on the page. The pictures were nearly all black and white, and were drawn in pencil or charcoal. The blacker the pictures were, the more poignant they would become. When I picked my pencil up it became a tool to illustrate an intensity that was building up like a volcano in my body. Sometimes I could draw and it was of no significance to me. Sometimes it meant more to the nurses and Dr Lynn, as it was telling them something even though I hadn't engaged with it. The drawings could be of significant tools that had been dangerous, such as razor blades, rope, sharps, hangings and symbols such as graves and crosses. Other times it could be big black clouds and parts of a body underneath them. Sometimes I added red to symbolise the cuts and the blood. At times they didn't mean anything and then it was as if somebody had pulled a switch. I did engage and in that split second I reacted and acted out. The impulsivity made it dangerous, as which picture, if any, would trigger a reaction was unpredictable, and so was the intensity.

***

Flashback:
I had reacted and I ran pushing open the heavy door leading to the staircase. I bounded up them and leapt onto a small ledge halfway up the stairs and level with the rooftop of an adjacent building. I crouched, panting, and then my adrenalin came into force and I turned looking through the slatted window to the rooftop that attracted me, but there was a considerable gap between the next building and the ledge I was on. A nurse appeared on the top of the next flight of stairs and he spoke with an urgent tone of voice. "Hey, you, get down from there!". I stared at him, feeling my heart pounding. Another nurse appeared next to him: a young girl with blonde hair. "Are you OK? Do you want some help?" She spoke gently and went to step towards the flight of steps leading down to my ledge. I turned and with incredible speed and force I smashed all the lower slats of glass within seconds. She jumped back, startled. I turned, staring at them and looking at the roof. I was contemplating jumping, but was not sure I would make the jump and it was a lethal drop if I didn't. Suddenly a voice I recognised came from the flight below me. "Bridget, what on earth are you doing? Get down from there at once!" I turned and Ruth had appeared, looking

quite angry. Her reaction spurred me on, and with a single blow I smashed the rest of the slats in the top window as if they were eggshells. The glass splintered and crashed to the floor below, and now I had enough room to jump. I raised my leg from my crouching position and as I jumped a hand grabbed my ankle and pulled me viciously off the ledge onto the cushion of bodies of nurses all rushing forward to grab me as I fell. I was marched back to my room, and Dr Lynn who had appeared out of nowhere and grabbed my leg, gave me a stern look and disappeared into the nurses' office to talk with them. I sat on my bed, staring stubbornly at the floor as the nurses grabbed my drawings and put them into the drawer. I felt shaken and bruised. I hadn't planned to even run. It had been irrational and impulsive, and if Dr Lynn hadn't grabbed me I might have leapt to my death. My life was balancing on delicate threads and how I was managed would determine whether I would survive or not.

**

As I reflected back, it became apparent how associations could change your view. Art used to be one of my favourite hobbies. As a teenager I would often be found with a sketchpad in my hand. Now when I think of art, my memory is of those horrific illustrations and the awful consequences of the drawings. I was lucky to have survived many times from acting out. Still being passionate about art, I hope that I will be able to replace these memories of more recent times, especially as Jo Jo is such an accomplished artist and just thinking of any of her drawings fills me with warmth that hopefully one day will eradicate the cold.

**

We watched Tee Jay play rugby, and my old teacher talked to me, asking whether either Tee Jay or Jo Jo liked art. "Jo Jo loves art, but unfortunately she didn't get on with the art teacher so changed subject." I spoke with genuine regret.

"That's a problem when there is only one teacher for a particular subject," my old teacher replied. I nodded. We both turned to look at the game as his grandson Ed scored a try. We clapped and stamped our feet to try to block out the cold wind blowing across the fields.

Later that day I was watching the television when again more news about Jimmy Savile was broadcast. When the first allegations about him and child abuse offences were shown, it had made me feel ill and had triggered a crisis. It brought back unwanted feelings with associations, and I had fallen into a pit of feeling unworthy, guilty and sick. Alongside this my stability had been threatened and I fought against the old feelings of wanting to self-harm and run away. After several years of moving forward with confidence and self-esteem, and moving to a more positive place in life, I felt I had fallen backwards into a pool of uncertainty. Once again I viewed everyone with trepidation, and felt that the whole world was an evil place to live in. I soon realised I was not alone, because I started to receive messages from other survivors who felt the same. Some of these survivors also relayed to me their fears for their children. They worried excessively if a similar event of abuse would happen to their child. Most parents are protective to their children but survivors of abuse are particularly concerned as they have experienced the dangers and are more sensitive to them than non-survivors. It was a subject that Dr Lynn had talked over with me consistently through our therapy sessions. He was concerned how I would handle my children reaching puberty. How I would handle them having a relationship, and if I could accept them having a relationship. He was concerned that I might inappropriately be too protective, and also concerned of the feelings and emotions that their actions would bring back to me. Although I denied that I would let my own past affect the way I felt about my children and being protective. I was relieved that we had covered the subject, as I could gain insight to the potential problems and hopefully manage the time when it came to the best of my capability.

I tried to share how I felt about Jimmy Savile when I saw Dr Lynn. I felt frustrated, completely mixed up, and in one sense I felt I had a private anger that was welling up inside me. I was uncertain why, but I felt it to be unfair that just as I was starting to gain ground and place my past behind me, the news and media about the case had sprung into action. Every day there seemed to be more news and unwanted triggers that sent me reeling. I was also saddened for the victims, and it angered me that according to the media there had been signs and signals that everything was not OK yet no one had done anything about it.

Dr Lynn was his normal pragmatic self. "It's not straightforward; the situation is complex. The survivors, as you know, may not have come forward for years as they were in denial. You also know from your private experience that people faced with adversity don't want to believe it or accept it. There are many reasons why this case is so complex." I took a deep breath and sighed. I knew he was talking sense, and that the situation was complicated. It didn't help as the whole thing had made me feel very sick, and I knew it had affected many survivors, causing some of them to have relapses. I also knew that most people felt sickened by it. Dr Lynn used the case to challenge my own thoughts on my past. I had never verbally admitted the harm or wrong the people had done to me. When he challenged me I would repeatedly tell him they loved and cared about me and that they had helped me, as it was easier for me to remember the good things that had happened and not the bad. I knew in my head that if a survivor told me the same about their experiences I would want to shout and tell them to wake up and see the damage that had been done. Dr Lynn challenged me again, and he used Jo Jo as an example. "So according to you the people in your past were

OK because although they fucked you and in some cases nearly killed you, it's OK because they were nice at times and were kind to you." It was a strong statement, and I flinched when he used the word 'fucked'. I never liked it, but I could understand why he used 'fucked', as the impact was direct and strong. He continued. "If Jo Jo came home and told you she had been fucked but the man was nice and gave her a cuddle, that would be alright?" He sounded cynical and I reacted.

"Of course it wouldn't be alright, but that's different."

"Why?" He looked straight at me as he asked.

"You know why: they were kind to me and they saved me from killing myself at times." My voice faltered because it seemed strange to me, but it was the truth at the time. I thought back...

***

Flashback:
It was nice for him to take the time out to try to help me find my biological mum. It seemed the most important thing in the world to me, and the fact that he had given me time off and helped me use his office to see the counsellor was nice. It was significant because besides Sandra he was the only other person in the whole world who cared about me finding my real mum. I loved my adoptive parents and saw them as my real parents, but I also had a deep-down yearning to find my biological mum. I couldn't ask my mum and dad, as they would immediately change the subject if I ever mentioned anything about my roots. I didn't want to hurt them, but seeing the relationship between them and my younger sister Denny and hearing the remarks about her resemblance to them tore at me, and it motivated me to find my mum. Sandra had been keen to help, and she had always emphasised the difference in how my parents treated my younger sister to how they treated me. Whether it was justified or not, I felt an emptiness and I wanted to find my mum. I didn't realise at the time just how serious my situation was or even acknowledge that anything was wrong. Already at the age of seventeen I had been groomed to such an extent by Sandra that when the bank manager first allowed me to use his office to see the counsellor and had asked me to stay behind so that he could help me with the information she was to leave me, I suspected nothing. Even when he had thrown me against the filing cabinets and had raped and abused me I had immediately suppressed it. I had clung onto the little piece of scrap paper that the counsellor had given to me and had treasured the writing that was so like mine on there. It had the words, 'I gave my baby away because I wanted her to have a better life than the one I could have given to her'. As my fingers touched the

146

paper, I felt I had at last come to a tiny step closer to finding my mum, and I had a link between her and myself. I had arrived home more worried about the excuse for being late, without giving away anything of looking for my biological mum, and also I had been desperate to get my skirt into the washing machine to hide all the blood that was on it. I had walked in and greeted my parents and we had tea together as if it had been a normal day at work. The next day I had been grateful to the bank manager as he again had asked me to stay behind where he could look up the address the counsellor had given me and see if we could find any trace of where my mum lived. He had given me a massive hug and promised me that we were a step closer in finding her. At the same time he had done similar actions, and it seemed strange but I had blocked it out. I could remember the hugs and the support, and looking the address up. It was nice that he could stop the intense desperation I had, even though at the time I hadn't realised I was desperate. He seemed to rescue me and make me feel better. He would ring me up and ask me to meet him, and I would make a false excuse to my parents and go. The awful feeling of despair and the intense feeling of the black and dark would stop when I saw him. He had a power over me that most people would not understand. I grew to love him, adore and worship him, and think that anything he did was OK. Yet at the same time I was being horrifically abused and it was as if I was under a spell. I at the same time was stuck because he would often mention he might tell my parents I was tracing my mum, and at other times threaten my little sister Denny's career as she also worked for the bank. Some of the abuse was so extreme: he used to strip me down in the car and hold the cigarette lighter to my private parts. He used to rape me when staff were in the neighbouring room and took the abuse to extreme levels, which became like a dare and a challenge. I look back and use those labels, but at the time it was as if none of the bad was happening and he was helping me. I became completely hooked on him, even to the extent that when his wife found out, I invited her over to my house when my mum and dad were out to explain that it wasn't how she thought it was. Even when I was explaining to her I was still in denial, because at another level it wasn't happening. Her response was to tell me to not let him know I had seen her and to report back to her. I did, as I was so happy that someone was helping me and it was as if my feelings were transferred to her as she had promised to help. It again was as if I was acting out on pieces of a jigsaw, but was not capable of piecing the whole thing together. My mind saw what it needed to see, not what was actually happening. The bank manager's wife met up with me a few times over the next couple of months and laughed that her husband did not know what she knew.

Again I was blind to the sickness of it all, as I had someone I could talk to and she seemed kind and praised me, telling me her boss knew my dad and he spoke about his middle daughter with pride. I had needed to hear this, as I always thought it was Denny they were proud of. It came to a pinnacle when out of the blue she demanded I leave his branch and work at another branch. I could not handle being parted from the branch, and one weekend on January 5th I trudged twenty miles in the pouring rain and ended up near their house. I was lost what to do, and took a whole bottle of paracetamol. I then became scared, as I hadn't passed out and was not thinking rationally. I rang the bank manager for help. His wife answered and I told her in desperation that I had swallowed a whole bottle of paracetamol and nothing had happened. She told me I hadn't taken enough and needed to get some more, and that I had to go to the chemist. I was in such a bad way that I followed her instructions and took another lot. I ended up having my stomach pumped at the LRI. Although my life was in danger for a few days, the medical professionals told me that I had only survived because I hadn't eaten, so it hadn't been absorbed into my body. Even then I still wanted to be with the bank manager and his wife. I needed help, but due to a young nurse telling me what to say to the routine psychiatrist so I would be OK, I was discharged. I returned to work after a week, much to the amazement of the bank manager. I unconsciously had again suppressed the bad and had only seen what to me was the good in life. I had felt that if I hadn't got the bank manager or Sandra I would be dead, as they both helped me and were kind to me.

***

Dr Lynn spoke quietly but with authority. "It was because of them you have so much damage."

"You still don't get it. They were really nice to me as well, and if the bank manager hadn't been so good when I needed it I would have been dead. He saved me from killing myself." I looked at Dr Lynn and felt frustrated because I could still feel how desperate I had felt and how the bank manager made the desperation disappear.

"So people who rape you, burn you and threaten you are nice people?" He looked at me seriously. "Come on, even you can't get out of this one."

"You just don't understand," I replied quietly.

"I do, and it's because they were so 'nice' to you as well that you are so fucked up."

I looked at him defiantly. "Yes, I might be, but I can't change how it happened just to suit you or change how I feel."

"That's the point. You are here to change and you must want to change," he said. He looked at his watch. "Right, we have to leave it there. Same time in two weeks." He stood up and I gathered my coat and bag and followed him out through the dark waiting room and building to outside.

When I left the sessions with Dr Lynn, they always challenged me, and as I drove home I was thinking of what he had said. I was of course against rape and abuse, and would have been horrified and upset if it had happened to anyone else. I would also be angry and want the abuser to be punished. Yet repeatedly when I was questioned about my past it was as if my mind had blocked and I could only remember the good. This was still a significant issue in child abuse, as many of the survivors suppressed the abuse and were then vulnerable for it to happen to them again. Because of the suppression and denial, people who may have been able to help couldn't because they were not aware, and the survivor continued to live under denial. Many people are unaware of how powerful the suppression and denial is, and blame the survivor for letting the abuse continue. Some people prefer not to believe the circumstances and others just think the survivor has made the situation up. The survivor is unconscious of the suppression and denial. It is a natural coping method, the brain protecting the mind from the trauma of the incidents. Child abuse is complex as when years later when the truth and trauma submerge, the people closest and who care about the survivor might then use denial for themselves to cope which again does not help the survivor, and again the survivor doesn't want to accept the truth.

I realised through messages from other survivors that sadly denial was a major problem for them too, as friends and family refused to accept and acknowledge their past. It brought additional hurt and misery to the survivor, and whereas they may have healed on a faster pathway they again were hit with pain and rejection. I could relate, as I had wrongly expected my family, my mum and sisters to empathise and make everything OK. Although Dr Lynn repeatedly explained to me that it was not going to happen, I still wanted it to, and it took many months for me to come to terms with the rejection and hurt. I could not understand how my mum could welcome my brother-in-law into her house and make him tea and talk to him as if nothing had happened when she knew he had abused me in the past. I could not understand why close relatives who found out said nothing to me. I wanted them to, as I needed the reassurance that people had cared what had happened, but it never came through the people who I thought loved me and were family and friends. Ironically it came from people who had never met me and had read my book and were horrified that it had happened. When I analyse this, it appears that the people who were close to me could not handle the hurt and pain, and consequently preferred not to mention it and to block it off. On the other hand, those who cared about what had happened through reading the book were safer to take the knowledge in as they didn't know me and could express their feelings. When Dr Lynn told me that child abuse was complex, it seemed that years of experience and knowledge were only just starting to sink in, and I was just on the tip of being able to understand the way people thought and behaved towards it. I was thankful that I had the support from my consultant, as although the abuse had happened years ago, the consequences and effect from it were still surfacing and he seemed to be the only person who I knew that cared about what had happened, what was still happening in my life and he also could explain to me why some of the consequences were so painful. I was fortunate that he was a clever dedicated man, passionate about his work, and he had a lot of patience as I sometimes took him to the limit.

***

The door opened, and as I waited in the corridor outside the outpatients room Dr Lynn walked through. After years of therapy I recognised the sound of his footsteps as he came down the stairs. The only time he had caught me out was when he had turned up for the session using the lift nearby, as he was on crutches and had his foot in plaster. This was a typical sign of his dedication to his job, as throughout the years of seeing him he had hardly missed a session.

"Let's face it: you are only helping me because you are paid to do it." I spoke with conviction as Dr Lynn was attempting to tell me that people did care and I was wrong in my beliefs.

"You are so fucking rude. Do you know that?" He spoke calmly and quietly. I felt guilty, yet it was what I believed at the time.

"I mean it with respect, but it's true," I replied.

Dr Lynn shook his head and smiled. "I know the next thing you will want me to do is kick and beat you up to prove that we are all the same... well, I am not going to do it." We both smiled as he often repeated this at different sessions. It wasn't the first time I had told him that he was only helping me because it was part of his job. I could nearly sense the resentment in him as I stated my convictions. I felt bad, as part of me wanted to believe people cared, but to me that would open the door on hurt and rejection. It was safer to believe the worst, then anything else that came was extra bonus. Dr Lynn had been seeing me since 1994, and it had taken seven years of his patience to help me recover to the stage where I could communicate a little more, to the extent in 2001 where I was admitted to the wards for more intense therapy. Once on the ward he also kept to his promise of seeing me every day and working hard with me to move me forward with my recovery, even when the two weeks' initial stay turned into a sectioning and eight months hospitalised. Although I was on level one the majority of the time, he allowed me to take walks with the appropriate nurses and understood my

150

fears of medication and need to be allowed outside. I had still been vulnerable on the wards and would rely heavily on his visits and those of Andrea, was my community psychiatric nurse. It was Dr Lynn who had persuaded me to stop seeing Sandra, and with Joseph's support we had cut her out of our lives. This had been extremely difficult for me, as to me I still loved and thought of her as a blend of a mother and sister. I had blocked out the fact that she had groomed me from the age of twelve and had abused me. I was still in a state of denial, to the extent where I had asked her to be a godparent to my children. It was Dr Lynn who had forced the issue and had taken the time to sit with both Joseph and me to explain the actions needed. When I had texted Sandra from my hospital bed to confront her, as I had been encouraged to do, her answer had been that I was already damaged before she had met me. This had enraged Andrea and the medical staff. At the time I was still too ill to take it all in. After the eight months of being in hospital, against all advice I went to see Sandra, and to take her a Christmas card.

***

"What do you want?" Sandra looked at me with disgust.

Her cold tone shook me and a tremor rippled through my body. I passed her the Christmas card. I still loved her and I wanted us to be friends.

"I needed to talk, to ask you… they told me you're a paedophile, that you didn't really love me?"

I hesitated, my voice shaking. I looked at her, imploring her to explain and tell me that they had it all wrong.

"I told you already. You were already damaged before we met. All I did was to love and look after you and this is how you repay me."

The door slammed in my face, and shaken but in a trance-like state I climbed back into my car to return home. My heart beat rapidly. I knew Joseph would be really angry if he knew I had been to see her, but I wanted to find out for myself. I felt at a loss because when Dr Lynn had told me to cut all ties with Sandra, it was a life-changing move. Over the last twenty years her family had been like a family to me. I had stayed with her relatives, been accepted as part of her family and her friends had become my friends. It was not only Sandra I was cutting off, but a massive segment of my social life.

***

It had been difficult, as paedophiles are clever at grooming and the attachment to them can be very strong. Even though they are abusing the person, the suppression and denial prevent the survivor perceiving the truth and understanding the need to break free.

151

My parents hated it when I first had an appointment with Dr Lynn; they had no idea why I needed to see him except that I had been referred after losing my memory from a car accident (although it was still arguable whether it had been intended for my car to break down or not). My parents had covered up when I had taken the overdose years ago. They had built on the diagnosis that I had a heart murmur and used that as the reason I had been admitted to the hospital when I had had my stomach pumped. Although I had attempted to tell my Mum about the bank manager years back, she had never taken it seriously or given it another thought. They never questioned me about seeing Dr Lynn, and I never gave an explanation. They had no idea of the abuse, and at that stage I hadn't acknowledged it either. When I did go into hospital in 2001 it was a couple of years after losing my dad, and my mum still didn't understand the full reasoning behind the admittance.

My best friend and her husband had no idea of the abuse either, so I was in the hospital with no support except from Joseph, who had his hands full with his business, Jo Jo and Tee Jay – both toddlers – and our animals. I relied on and turned to Dr Lynn and Andrea for my way out to recovery. I made some good friends with many of the nurses, yet still respected their professional boundaries.

***

On the ward it was easy to become institutionalised, and Dr Lynn would do his best to warn me and protect me from some of the patients, as did some of the nurses. One nurse warned me whilst I was self-harming to be careful because another patient had MRSA and how dangerous it could be. She did break the confidentiality of the elderly patient, but I had appreciated the advice and kept my distance, and it also made me think whilst I was cutting – but unfortunately it didn't stop me. I had felt intense despair without realising it, and at times I was unfair to Dr Lynn, as after he had spoken to me in my room I would be desperate for him not to go and would stand across the door to stop him leaving.

***

Flashback:
"Don't do that, Bridge." His six-foot-seven frame filled his suit and blocked the sunlight seeping through the window, and I glanced up at him. I couldn't speak; I didn't want him to go. I looked up at him, hand clenched on the door handle keeping the door closed. He leaned forward to try to get to the handle and I flinched and he stepped back again. "Bridge," he pleaded.
I stared at him forlornly. I was desperate. "Bridge, please don't do this." He looked at me and I regretfully stood aside to let him go. He beckoned a nurse into my room as he turned to walk up the corridor. "I'll see you tomorrow." He smiled at me and I turned to sit on my bed. He would arrive at any time and some days it was

frustrating, as I wanted to go out but was scared of missing his visit. I got into a habit of ringing Mary, his secretary, to find out what time he would be coming. She was great with me and would often tell me when she thought he'd be down on the ward.

"Bridge, quick, quick!" Rita my nurse had just told me it was OK to put my shorts on as it was a really warm day, and I was changing when she heard the familiar footsteps coming up the ward corridor. "Quick, quick!" She was flustered as we saw his huge figure against the glass window and she suddenly pushed against the door. I saw it try to open and shut again as she was pushing her weight on it. I zipped up my shorts and pulled my T-shirt over just in time as Dr Lynn walked in. "What's going on?" he asked, looking at her. She didn't respond as she walked out giggling and I stemmed a laugh, trying to look at him seriously as he sat down to talk. Another time he would place the odd piece into a jigsaw I was completing as he talked to me.

I appreciated his visits and the work he and Andrea were doing with me, and I tried to respect them and do my best, but I was also very ill and still acted out irrationally and impulsively. One day I was so worked up after waiting for a routine ward round to finish that when they both came into my room to talk to me I stood up, pacing the room as they both sat there. Andrea lost her patience and told me to sit down. I responded like a little kid, slamming the wardrobe door back and forth on the wall and making myself jump at the sound it made. I was upset, and the intensity of my despair was growing. Dr Lynn sat with his long legs stretched out, waiting calmly for me to settle down. I didn't, suddenly picked up my television and threw it across the room. Andrea jumped and reacted angrily. Dr Lynn hadn't flinched. The nurses came rushing in. "Bridge, you will have to come out whilst they clear up." Dr Lynn still spoke calmly and I walked out of my room with them. I stood watching the nurses clear my television up, part of me really upset as it had been a present from Sandra and it had sentimental value. The nurses soon took the last pieces and the room was clear again. I suddenly realised that no one was monitoring me and that the nearest nurse was across the room. I sprinted to my room and grabbed a mug off the side of the sink, smashing it on the side. I aimed for the jugular vein on my neck and slashed as hard as I could. I saw the blood on the floor and before I could do anything else I was taken down by a group of nurses. I struggled to retain my grip on the mug, but it was knocked out of reach. Dr Lynn sat on my bed, looking down at me, and as I pulled my hand away from my neck it was dripping with blood. I saw Dr Lynn looking at it and he now moved quickly towards me to inspect the damage. I had just missed my jugular vein but had cut part of my ear lobe badly. I was patched up with sterile strips holding my ear together and a bandage around my neck. I was muttering away non-stop. "I wish you were all dogs, then I would be safe. Dogs don't hurt, do they?" The nurses spoke softly and they were nice whilst Dr Lynn hovered anxiously directing the nurses to make sure they did the best possible job of patching me up to minimise scarring.

***

I was fortunate to have Dr Lynn as my consultant, as I believed another consultant may have drugged me or sent me to seclusion. He was genuinely concerned and attempted to understand why I did what I did. I hadn't planned to act out, and it was as much a surprise to me as it was the nurses. I also regretted my actions sometimes, especially as I smashed around seventeen windows during my stays. One day on an outpatient visit to see Andrea I was waiting upstairs as usual when a workman who was replacing the windows decided to chat to me.

"Feel that," he said, and he passed me a small piece of glass that was about an inch square.

I fingered it, feeling the thickness. "Hmm," I answered back, not really knowing what to say to him.

"See this." He gestured to the window where he had just replaced the glass. "I am having to replace all these because the authority think they may be sued."

"Why?" I asked.

He continued even though I had interrupted him. "A patient here went through seventeen windows. Must have been right screwed up, but they think they may get sued so have had instructions to replace them all. This new glass will not shatter even if a bomb went off." I nodded and raised my eyebrows. Just then Andrea appeared and I beckoned her over.

"Guess what," I said with a wink. "This guy has been instructed to replace all the windows because they had a patient here who smashed seventeen. Imagine that! And they are worried they might sue."

"That's right," said the guy, again raising his eyebrows as he passed the one-inch square bit to Andrea. "Feel that. Tough, isn't it?" Andrea fought back her smile and nodded. She beckoned me to follow her and I nodded at the guy as I followed her through to the room. Once inside we both started laughing.

"He would have died if he had known it was you," Andrea said. I laughed, as I also found it quite amusing.

"I would never sue. I felt bad that I had damaged them. I was offered the chance of asking for money for my bag of clothes I had stolen when I was sent to the high security unit, but I refused because I felt guilty about all the windows I had broken," I told Andrea. She was still laughing and we settled down to continue with the therapy.

***

When I started to be able to communicate a little more with Dr Lynn, he changed the appointments from seeing me weekly to seeing him fortnightly. In between these appointments I had to see different doctors in his team. I roughly spent six months seeing each one, as they were on a time schedule for the different departments in their training. I was very wary at first, but managed to get on well with some of them. One doctor from New Zealand, Darren Malone, returned back there, and I managed to send him a copy of my first book. Another doctor, who I nicknamed Pingu after the TV penguin, was brilliant, and he managed to build my self-esteem very well. I learned to gradually trust them a little, but I always hated the farewells and had a job to manage them. Dr Lynn thought meeting different people was good for me, as it would prove to me that not everyone was out to hurt me. Even to this day I still hate saying goodbye to people. If my parents ever went on holiday I would love to pick them up at the airport but would refuse to take them. I also got on well with many of the nurses, and after spending nearly four years in hospital knew quite a few of them very well. I was even invited to a staff party, but declined for several reasons.

CHAPTER TWENTY-ONE – GOODBYE TO A GEM

It was the beginning of December 2012, and I walked up to the local hospital from the car park. I had been coming to see Dr Stirton for the last ten years, and she had been a massive support for both of the children. Jo Jo had unfortunately been having breathing problems of late and we were not sure if it was panic attacks or exercise-induced asthma. It was complex and we had been discussing whether CBT would help. At the present time Jo Jo was seeing a physiotherapist, who seemed to be helping her build her confidence and manage the problems a little better. Dr Stirton had also helped me to support Tee Jay, who with his specific learning difficulties and dyslexia had to fight for·the correct support at school. He had been referred to Dr Stirton in the past for anxiety caused by a special needs teacher refusing to give the correct medical breaks when needed. The situation had escalated to Tee Jay becoming quite ill, but thanks to the brilliant therapy by Dr Stirton and her team and moving to his next school, Tee Jay had rebuilt his confidence. Tee Jay had a Special Educational Needs Certificate, and the school was not fulfilling the statement to the appropriate requirements, and Dr Stirton had been a terrific support in many ways. She had helped me manage the children, advising me what to do in specific circumstances, attending some of the reviews, and she had also backed up my medical support as it was important that I managed my health needs to be able to be as good a mum as possible for the children. I put the children first and had often been praised for the way I managed to cope with some of the difficult situations that occurred. Now after a period of ten years of support, I was saying goodbye, as Dr Stirton was leaving the service. I felt nothing but gratitude and appreciation for the time she had given me, and as I walked through the doors for the appointment, I felt a wave of sadness overcome me as she had been a key figure in helping me to gain my confidence. She had also encouraged me so much in my final years of taking my psychology degree and had told me to concentrate hard on it in the last year.

I sat in the empty waiting room and stared at the corkboard on the wall. Tee Jay's drawing from a few years back was still pinned up, and he would have laughed if he had seen it. I hadn't had to wait long before Dr Stirton popped her head around the door and invited me to the consulting room. I followed her. She was a petite lady with dark short hair, glasses and a beaming smile.

"And how are things?" she asked, pen and pad ready as I started to reply.

"Well, Jo Jo saw the physiotherapist…"

I told her about both of the kids and how life was at home. We also talked about Dr Lynn as Dr Stirton had known him for many years, and because I had been seeing both of them for different reasons they had communicated well. They both seemed to have a good professional mutual respect for each other, and as the clock showed half past three I knew it was time to go. Dr Stirton stood up. She wasn't very tall, but her presence was felt through the respect people had for her.

"Can I give you a hug?" she asked.

I nodded, and as we hugged she said, "I want to give you one more piece of advice." I looked at her; she was smiling. "Don't look so worried, it isn't bad." She laughed, and I laughed too, still apprehensive.

"You have it, you have it all. Just believe in yourself," she said.

I nodded. "Thank you, and thank you for believing in me." I hugged her again.

"Tell Jo Jo and Tee Jay to look after themselves."

"I will do, and thank you for everything."

She smiled as she held the door open for me and I walked back out.

I knew that I had been privileged to have seen Dr Stirton and received her support for the length of time I had it for, and I hoped that I had put the advice to good use. I also hoped that she had recognised how much her support had been appreciated. The rest of the month flew by and I realised I would miss her.

It was coming up to Christmas and I was wrapping the presents. I had left it to the last minute and was trying to wrap them before the kids broke up from school. I wasn't the neatest of wrappers, and saw it as a chore rather than a gesture of love and thanksgiving. The Sellotape covered tears and the 'Love from Santa' tags all matched. I was glad when I had finished, as it was time-consuming and I knew I had to tidy the house before my mum came. However tidy it was, Mum would always have to tidy more and we always knew when she had visited as the tea towels were neatly folded into regimental folds instead of stuffed in the drawer.

Mum was in her eighties now, and liked routine, which meant meals a lot earlier than we would normally have and a biscuit with her cup of tea, and so on. Joseph got told off for not warming the plates beforehand as he served up a fantastic Christmas dinner, and I sent him a warning glance as I could see he was about to retaliate. He bit his lip walking into the kitchen to fetch the rest of the meal. We celebrated and pulled the crackers and laughed at the cats as they played with some of the toys that fell onto the floor. After dinner we watched television and opened more presents. The kids, all grown up, had bought their own presents for us, and it was the special way they brought them to us that touched my heart and embedded deep into my mind. The smile they had on their faces as they passed the presents over was sensitive, and I could tell it meant a lot to them how we reacted. Jo Jo had bought some fruit-scented bath gel, a hoodie, and a special Mum mug, and Tee Jay had bought me some chocolates and a pen. They had then both contributed in buying a large diabetic selection of chocolates. "Come here, both of you," I said as I stood up and gave Jo Jo a massive hug and kiss and Tee Jay leaned over and hugged me hard too. "Love you both." I smiled at them.

"Love you too." We all laughed as they had said it together. Joseph smiled on as he unwrapped a top from Jo Jo and a T-shirt from Tee Jay. Joseph had bought a few selective presents, wrapping them carefully using ribbons and nice paper. They looked lovely. His small messages seemed more passionate as they were written in French and seemed to carry significant weight. Mum was impressed, as he had bought her a lovely plant and some chocolates and soaps. The dogs enjoyed their treats out of their stockings and the cats seemed happier playing with the empty boxes and paper then anything else. Tee Jay had been out to the paddock and all the animals had been given extra straw, hay and special vegetable treats to mark the day.

Mum stayed over on Boxing Day and then returned home before going to visit Denny. We had a couple of lazy days and I started to get to know my iPad better. Facebook had introduced me to so many special people, whatever the media threw at it, and I knew I would be always grateful. One of the special people it had introduced me to was my biological sister called Angie. She and I had sent messages a few times and although we had never met we were both amazed at how much we had in common. We both loved animals, the outdoors, bird-watching and similar television programmes amongst many other things. Although our values and principles may have differed to some degree, we were very similar. We also had similar health ailments and as neither of us smoked, used drugs, or drank heavily, it would seem the ailments were similar because of the genetic background. We emailed and messaged quite a bit and Angie offered to come and see me. I had never met her and had agreed that we would meet. However, when it came to actually doing it, I backed out. I still question myself why, as on the one hand I could be missing out on a special relationship, yet on the other I so valued that we had become friends and I think part of me was scared that something could go wrong. I think my past still clouded some of my decisions, and it was an area that I had to work on. Deep down I had thought that this was down to trust, but I think I trusted Angie – it was more of a case of being scared of being hurt and it was the building of the relationship that I didn't trust and I didn't want to ruin any part of the special relationship I had already. I hoped that Angie would understand this, and I think she did, because it is something like three years later and we are still communicating and love each other at our own levels and understanding. It was also complicated as I didn't want to hurt my mum or sisters, and I wasn't sure if Denny would understand completely or not. My mum, because of her age, was harder to talk to. It was as if she was becoming more set in her state of mind and less open to any additional influences.

Angie and I looked like sisters, and on our mum's side we all had high cheekbones and similar facial features. I searched Angie's friends and found some of my biological relatives. I was naturally curious. Jo Jo told me off for stalking, and in one way I felt a bit guilty but I felt justified as they were related and if their privacy settings had allowed me to look, well, so be it.

Dr Lynn seemed to be rather dubious about Facebook and would often comment, "In the real world…" I knew what he meant, but in one way when I saw him it seemed to be outside the real world. I would enter the room with him and some of the conversations we had were so private I knew that they would never be issues I would repeat with anyone else. It had taken me years and years to reach this stage of confidence, and although I had reached it with Dr Lynn I still only trusted a handful of people who I could confide in. I talked certain things through with friends, but at a much lighter level. At home I would just get on with things as many people do, but it was nice to be able to have an outlet when I needed it.

As Jo Jo and Tee Jay were growing up I found that I could talk more and more to them, but I was still very aware they were children and to me it was vital that they enjoyed their childhood and had no extra responsibilities that could burden or spoil their maturity. At the same time it became apparent that they grew to understand more, and there became a balance of being open and honest and although the protection level decreased, I was still aware that they were children Dr Lynn would ask me how the children were doing, and he was very astute about my emotions as Jo Jo reached puberty in the earlier years.

***

"Do you want Jo Jo to have a boyfriend?" Dr Lynn waited, as there was a silence.

"Of course I do," I replied.

"Will you feel protective?"

"Every mother would feel protective, and I am no different."

"What will you do if she wants to have sex?"

The question actually made me feel ill, as my daughter was still very young and it wasn't a subject that I had thought about a lot. "I am still pretty old-fashioned, but it would depend on her age and it would depend on the circumstances. At the end of the day I want my daughter to be happy, but of course I would want to protect her and guide her. Jo Jo is very sensible, and I think when she reaches the appropriate age she will be a very good judge of what she wants."

"Will you resent it if she is having a happy sexual relationship?"

"Of course I wouldn't."

"What happens if her boyfriend or partner has sex with her and she didn't want it? Would you feel that was wrong? Would you be upset?" Again there was a silence, as I felt annoyed at the questions and after several sessions like this I knew where it was leading.

"Of course I would be upset," I replied indignantly.

"Why would you get upset for your daughter, but not upset at your own past? How is it wrong for her to be raped, but not wrong when you were?" I jumped as he mentioned the word 'raped', and my arms flung back as if someone had given me an electric shock. I quickly gathered myself and answered back. "It's different, you know it is."

"Explain."

"You don't understand. It's just different." Already my mind had started to block and I struggled with my words. As I was talking to him I was thinking of the desperation I had been in and how in my past the people who he allegedly called rapists would comfort me and hug me and help me. I could still feel the intensity of how I thought at the time they were rescuing me. Dr Lynn sighed and I shrugged my shoulders. It was so hard to explain that when I remembered back it was as if I had invisible barriers. It was as if I was in a trance, so it was like looking and knowing but not engaging. I read this, and think I have contradicted myself, as half of me has just described the despair I could remember, and the removal of it as they hugged me, and then as he asks me to remember the whole picture I couldn't. It was as if it was to someone else. Dr Lynn often told me I would split and that to be well I had to piece the whole thing together.

***

My children were growing up fast, and I cared about how they enjoyed their life. As I write this I feel guilty because despite of the bad things that happened to me, I still felt extremely lucky. I still love my adoptive parents and to me they are my mum and dad. I was devastated when I lost my dad in 1999 and I love him just as much to this day. I look back at some of the decisions he made when I was suffering and don't agree with all of them, but to be fair he didn't know or understand what I was going through. How could he when I was still in denial and I didn't know myself? The same goes for my mum. I remember back and I think, when I took the overdose, if it had been my children I would have wanted to know much more about how, what, why, etc. Yet at the time my parents thought it was because of a transfer in the bank to another branch. The bank manager and his wife had told them this, and it was true as I didn't want to move. People can be quick to judge, but until you have been in the same situation it is hard to have a fair opinion. Everyone is unique and each circumstance individual. My only 'ifs' are when

I told my mum about the bank manager and her response was for me not to tell my dad. I wish she had acted, but I hadn't chased her either. I was also in denial so although I told my Mum about the bank manager, I may not have used strong enough words.Then again she could have been worried about what dad would do, or what effect it had on him, or what he might have said to me. I still don't know. The only other time was when I told my dad I had been to the police about my brother-in-law harassing me, and instead of backing me up he told me he was ashamed of me. I think this was from his upbringing and his generation where reputation and what others would think was all-important. Overall our family had a good home, a decent upbringing, and we were loved. Somehow along the way I had become introverted and lost. I ask whether it was because I was adopted, whether it was because I was the middle child, or because my friends were not always available. I now believe it was a combination of all of this: my genetics, the circumstances and also fate. I was vulnerable and unlucky enough to meet the wrong people. So many people misunderstand why victims of child abuse don't ask for help or stop what is happening. They are also quick to judge and blame the people around. It is wrong to do so, as child abuse is complicated due to the denial and suppression.

CHAPTER TWENTY-TWO – THE CHALLENGE

"Come on!" I shouted to the kids. They were both coming with me to the shopping precinct, where I was dropping them off on my way to the hospital. First we called in to see Mum, and she had left the door on the latch as she was expecting us.

"Alright?" I asked, as she looked pale.

"Not been good, but I am OK," Mum said. "Hello, darling, I'll have my hug then." Jo Jo gave her a big hug, and she turned to Tee Jay who bent down to give her a hug too. She laughed as she looked up to him. "Am I shrinking, or are you growing?" Tee Jay grinned at her. "Go on with you." Mum laughed and poured the tea and we followed her through to the lounge. Lottie, her little Russian terrier, followed and jumped onto Mum's knee before she had sat down properly. The kids went into the other room, each texting on their phones. I sipped my tea and listened as Mum told me where she was going with the volunteer group and what the meal was like in the pub the week before. I then sat for ten minutes listening to her go on about her hairdresser's kitchen and all the faults and setbacks she had suffered. It was twenty minutes later that, as Mum still talked about it, I changed the subject. It was obviously on my Mum's mind, but I was more interested in what Mum was doing for the week than in cracks in sinks and faults in oven doors. At half past nine we had to move as we had thirty minutes to get across town to the hospital and drop the kids off on the way. We all hugged my mum and I told her I would see her soon. She waved to us from her porch and I flicked the indicators on my car as I drove down her driveway. The kids waved like mad to her. I dropped them off in Thurmaston and told them I would be there around 11.30am. At the hospital I managed to park easily and after paying my £2.50 I walked through to the reception, as I had done for the last nineteen years, and stood in the corridor. It was quite sad standing on the first floor alone, as some of the hospital wards had already moved to the other hospital and people who I had got to know over the years had left. It wasn't long before I heard Dr Lynn's footsteps and he walked through the door. I waited as he unlocked the Outpatients door, and walked after him through the dark empty waiting area into the consulting room. I sat down and placed my coat and bag onto the vacant chair. Dr Lynn sat down and looked across to me. We sat in silence as we always did, yet this time he broke the silence, which was rare. "I have something to tell you." My heart started to race, as my gut instinct told me something was wrong. "I am leaving in May and your therapy will stop and you won't be seeing anyone else."

My arms flung aside again involuntarily, and as I tried to stop the room from reeling I sat in silence. I felt ill, sick and scared. Waves of despair tore through my body, and I stared at the window, every sense of my body telling me to go through it. I sat gripping my chair, telling myself this wasn't happening. Dr Lynn sat back and observed me. I sat feeling the tremors ripple through my body. It was as if my world had ended. People would condemn me for feeling this, and I condemned myself as I loved my children and family, but I felt like a diver deep down under the sea who had just had their oxygen tank emptied and still had to swim further than possible. I stared at Dr Lynn and he stared at me. The rest of the session was in silence, and forty-five minutes later I rose to go. I was like a zombie. "Two weeks." His words echoed, ringing around my head. I tried to switch to focus on picking up the kids, knowing I had a fight to stop tears rising. On my way out I bumped into Ruth, who I hadn't seen for years. "Hello, how are you doing?" she asked as we gave each other a bear hug. I liked Ruth. She had been one of the best nurses who looked after me. She looked older, as it was twelve years on since I first saw her in my hospital room. "Fine. I am just in shock as Trevor has just told me his news after nineteen years of seeing him." My voice shook as I told her and she smiled at me.

"Well, you have five months to get used to it." I smiled and hugged her goodbye. I made my way to the car. I drove quickly and once I was in the country lanes where I could see well ahead that there was no traffic I put my foot down to rid myself of the frustration. It was not the same feeling in an automatic car, as with manual gears I could ride and feel the speed, but it helped a little. Once in the built-up areas I slowed down and caught sight of the kids waiting at the side of the pavement. I grinned at them as they jumped in. "Had a good morning?" I asked.

"OK," said Jo Jo, and she pulled out her shopping to show me what she had bought.

"Alright?" I asked Tee Jay who was in the back. He nodded and smiled at me through the mirror. I took the carriageway as I wanted to get back quicker, and once home the kids disappeared into their bedrooms and I went into mine to get changed. I was just coming down when Jo Jo walked in.

"What's the matter, Mum?"

Shocked, I turned around to look at her. I had always managed to mask my feelings and obviously hadn't done a good job this time.

"I am OK. I just received a shock: Dr Lynn is leaving and it's natural that after nearly twenty years of support I feel a bit shocked and very sad." Jo Jo walked up to me and we hugged, and I felt a little better as I felt her arms around me. She stayed silent and hugged me again tighter. I felt guilty, as I knew she had missed me when I spent the four years in and out of hospital and I didn't want her to worry. "At least I won't have to travel all the way into Leicester, or save my 50p and £1 coins for the car park fees." I grinned at her. "Come on, I want a cup of tea. I'll be fine. It was just a shock." She smiled at me and returned to her room. I went downstairs, pondering on how grown-up she had become and also how astute.

Tee Jay came up to me about ten minutes later and gave me a hug. "What's that for?" I laughed and tried to tickle him. He jumped aside and rugby-tackled me, and we had a rough-and-tumble in the kitchen. I already knew deep down that Jo Jo must have talked to him. "It will be OK, Mum," he said quietly. It nearly set me off and I turned and he held me tight. "I'm fine, honestly, Tee. It's just a shock. Imagine twenty years of seeing someone week in week out for most of it. I just need time to adjust. It will be like losing a best friend, but I will be OK." Tee Jay nodded and he grabbed a biscuit from the tin.

"I am going into the paddock, see you later." He walked out and I sipped my tea thinking what great kids I had. The feeling of despair would not lift, and I couldn't focus to watch television, read a book or do anything else. I existed as a shell. I snapped at Joseph and I went to bed early. When I woke up in the mornings it was with that sick feeling when you know something is wrong. The appointments with Dr Lynn changed from a target that I had looked forward to, to an appointment that I dreaded. I thought about what I wanted to ask him and I sent him an email criticising the way he had told me. 'You could have said, 'Hey Bridget, I have something sad to tell you, but don't worry I will make sure that you still have the necessary support. I am leaving in May but I will give all your details to'…'

This would have still been a massive shock but it would not have left me so scared and frightened. I talked it over with Dr Dhanji. As I sat in her room I couldn't speak, and when she asked me if I was OK, I looked away as I had tears in my eyes. "Dr Lynn is leaving." It came out as a mumble.

"Well, we knew he would leave at some point, but don't worry, you will still have support." She smiled at me, her long dark hair dropping forward as she leaned towards me.

"I won't, though. He said that my therapy is ending and I will not be seeing anyone else. I don't want to see anyone else but it would have been nice to have the choice. I have worked hard towards my goal and he admitted I was 6/8 through. I feel let down. I feel like I have worked hard to build a house and he has left the roof off." I sat back. I felt angry and let down. I continued.

"I honestly feel like he is one of the people in my past, I have trusted him and he has let me down." A silence hit the room. I continued. "I have had his support for twenty years and Dr Stirton's for the last ten years. She has just left and I am still recovering from that. After twenty years of regular support I just can't go to nothing. The pressure is enormous." My voice cracked and I sat back. I was shaking and I felt bad. "I wouldn't mind, but he admitted I was three quarters through my therapy, so why not let me finish it?" Another silence as Dr Dhanji let me get grips with myself.

"I shall write to him," she replied.

I shook my head and spoke up. "No, please, I need to talk to him again and find out what is happening. It was too much of a shock before." I looked at her and she nodded in agreement.

The next time I went to see Dr Lynn, I found it nearly impossible to stay in the same room. He had been so kind to me that it hurt knowing I would not have that support.

"How will you cope? What will you do?" he asked me.

"What's the point of asking me?" I replied. "In a few months' time you won't want to know as you won't be paid for it."

"Fuck off," he retorted.

I leaned back in my chair.

"You can be so rude ,do you know that?" he added.

I looked at the ground. I was upset and I knew I had been rude, because deep down I knew he cared a lot, but I was hurting so badly. He looked at me and it hurt so much I grabbed my coat and bag and walked out. I nearly ran across the empty waiting room and opened the security door and ran into the corridor. There I stared at a cover of my book, *A Fine Line*, with an endorsement from all the medical professionals. I had been fortunate that the Trust had given me permission to place information about my book on the walls. I stared, thinking of all the support and all the friends I had made at the hospital over the twenty years. This seemed like a nightmare that I was living through and didn't want to happen. I went to walk out and then realised that I would be so full of frustration that I wouldn't be able to cope for the next two weeks. I turned and pulled the door handle to go back in. It wouldn't open; it was locked. 'Shit,' I said to myself under my breath. I stood there for ten minutes cursing once again my impulsivity. I waited and after a few minutes Dr Lynn appeared. He opened the door. "Do you want to come back in?" I nodded and followed his tall figure back across the waiting room to the consulting room. He held the door open for me and I slunk in as meek as a lamb. I sat feeling low.

"If you cared about me, you would make sure I had someone to contact even just in case of an emergency. You could have told me in a nicer way." I sat looking at the floor.

"There is no one, Bridge, and you know everything there is to know. Part of your recovery will be the working it out for yourself."

"But what if I had a crisis?"

"Dr Dhanji would refer you through the system like everyone else."

"But it seems daft when I already know most of the team to be referred to someone new."

"There is hardly any of the team left," he replied, and again there was an awkward silence.

I still felt upset and there was so much I wanted to ask but I was bottled up and I couldn't speak. The rest of the session was spent in silence and I rose to follow him out after he had again told me the next appointment time.

I drove home with mixed feelings, knowing how fortunate I had been to have received the support, yet part of me now wished I had not become so dependent. I still felt betrayed. Years back, I had worried about the leaving time, but had always believed I would either have been fully recovered or would have been referred to somebody else.

There was nothing for it but to get on with life, yet the next few weeks all I could think about was the time I had spent in hospital.

***

People think that when you get admitted into a psycho unit you become 'one of them'. Yet rationally many people didn't know that you had been receiving treatment and up to that time you were still unclassed. At what point does a person's view of you change from being unclassed to 'one of them'? Different people are bound to label by various definitions, some just because you have walked through the door of a psychiatric unit, others from behaviour...

When I walked through the door of the psychiatric unit I hadn't given it a thought that I would become 'one of them'. To me I was still me, and I was being referred because Dr Lynn thought it was necessary for me to talk about my past. At no stage had I thought of myself as being ill, although I knew I was suicidal and had started to cut just before going into hospital because I had been scared of the unknown. I had been told my stay would be for two weeks and although I was terrified and had nearly backed out of being an inpatient on the day of arrival I hadn't thought any of it through. My main concerns at the time were if the children would be looked after OK, if Tee Jay would be accepted at the day-care nursery still in nappies, and that the dogs and rest of the animals would be looked after. Joseph and I at the time never dreamed that the two weeks would turn into a sectioning and stay of eight months followed by an intermittent stay of a total of four years.

As I entered the ward, which was mainly for the elderly with a few of Dr Lynn's patients, it reminded me of an old people's home where I had helped out as a kid. The few younger people that were there seemed to be more of 'one of them', as some of the elderly patients' behaviour seemed to be acceptable because of their age. One of the younger patients soon made herself known to me and although many people might have found my actions

166

of self-harm, to which I never gave a second though, shocking, this patient's actions shocked and scared me.

She confided in me after I had been in there for a while.

"Hello, can I come in?" I looked up at the sound of knocking to see an attractive West Indian girl introducing herself. I warmed to her straightaway, as she was smiling and laughing. She was dressed in a T-shirt, jeans and a cardigan, and I guessed her to be in her twenties. "I am Kelly. Are you with him as well then?" she asked.

I nodded as I had seen Dr Lynn visit her. "Do you want a drink? I'll go and make one." I again nodded and she disappeared. I was relieved she hadn't asked me too much. It was to be some time later that she became friends and asked me to listen to a tape recording she had been asked to make. I found this uncomfortable and an invasion of her privacy, but she pleaded with me and told me I would understand her more. I listened but kept the information at a distance because it was the only way I could cope with it. I think I helped her more by just being there and being someone who she could talk to and have a laugh with than anything else. The tape shocked me, as I couldn't believe a dad could do those things, especially to his own daughter.

Kelly started to reveal more and more of her problems. One day she came into my room and as she sat down, pulled a shopping bag from her larger bag. "Can you do me a big favour?" she whispered as there was a nurse at the door reading a magazine. She quickly put the bag back into her bag, pointing at it.

"What?" I asked, having no idea what she was going to say.

"Can you look after this for me? They won't suspect you, as you only cut." I grimaced at this, not liking to be reminded and it sounded sick the way she had said it.

"What is it?" I peered into her bag.

"Bleach," she replied.

"Bleach, why?" I was still none the wiser.

"I use it a lot," she said.

"It's not that dirty, is it? I don't go into your ward. I know it smells sometimes." I said it quietly as I knew some of the oldest occupants often had accidents and although the nurses seemed to be efficient, there was always a distinctive aroma in the mornings when they changed the sheets. Kelly suddenly started to laugh. She laughed so much she was rolling about holding her stomach. She made me laugh too, although I had no idea what she was laughing at. We both had tears in our eyes.

"What? What have I said?" I asked her, wiping my eyes.

"It's not for the tables, you idiot. It's for me," Kelly answered.

"Shit, you don't drink it? You'd be dead!" I nearly shouted it out.

"Sssh." She gestured, reminding me of the nurse at the door.

"What do you do with it?" I asked, but I didn't really want to know. Yet I did.

"I rub my arms with it, I wipe it on me until I burn." She rolled her sleeve up and I felt sick as I looked at her burnt and scarred arms. I didn't judge, as she must have been in so much distress to take such an action to take the distress away.

"I can't do it," I replied quietly. She looked at me, shocked. "Sorry, Kelly, as much as I want to support you, I wouldn't be a real friend if I kept that for you. I want you to stop, but I understand why you do it. I just can't help you to hurt yourself." She grabbed the bag and stormed out of my room. I sat on my bed thinking about what I'd seen and wondering if different brands of bleach did more damage. My thoughts were sick, and soon I jumped off my bed to make a drink and to divert myself.

It was to be a day or so later that Kelly reappeared at my door. "Can I come in?" she asked.

"Of course you can." I smiled at her and she came in and sat down.

"I just wanted to say 'bye."

"What do you mean, 'bye?" I asked.

"I am being discharged. I shall be off in the next hour." She got up again. "You take care." And she walked out. I sat on my bed feeling upset and bewildered. How could she be discharged when she was doing awful things like burning herself? I was really upset by the time Dr Lynn came to visit me.

"How can you let her go? She needs help."

He looked at me. "None of your business."

"It is. She's my friend."

"Not really. Look, Bridge, I can only do so much, and if people don't want to help themselves, eventually I have no choice. If someone wants to kill themselves, they will. We can only do so much here. We have to help those who want to help themselves."

I remained silent. It seemed sad, but I could see where he was coming from.

"Now, let's concentrate on you." His tall frame leaned over as he started to explain what we were going to do next…

Another patient shocked me in a completely different way. She was a very well-spoken lady and I guessed she was in her early seventies. I was lying on my bed drawing a picture when I heard, "Please don't do that, Esther." I recognised the voice of Louise, one of the staff nurses, and the giggle of one of the trainees. "Sssh!" came a reprimand from Louise. "Esther." This time Louise sounded stern and I couldn't help but wonder what Esther was doing. I soon found out the next day: as I was coming out of the ward kitchen, Esther was walking down the corridor towards the reception stark naked and was masturbating. There was a startled gasp from Mustafa, a Muslim nurse. He had already grabbed a towel and running up to Esther had tried to cover her front as he led her back to the ward. A stifled ripple of laughter surrounded the room, but more people looked to the floor than laughed out loud. "Fucking hell. Who was that?" one of the new male patients shouted out. No one answered, as everyone was still shocked. After that incident I could never look at Esther, however charming and well spoken she was, without remembering the event.

One day, not long after I had been sectioned for running off the ward and cutting, Dr Lynn had just finished talking to me and was on his way out. I ran after him, and caught off his guard he leaned back against the wall. "What are you doing, Bridge?" He half laughed, and amused, he had glanced towards the nurse's room where Ruth was looking out through the glass window at us laughing. Standing on my tiptoes I had reached up, pinning Dr Lynn's arms against the corridor wall. "If I am not going anywhere, neither are you." I had said it determinedly and quickly. Dr Lynn laughed, but looked embarrassed. Ruth came running up. She was laughing so much she was nearly crying. "Come on, Bridge, put him down." I stepped back reluctantly and meekly. Once again I had acted out impulsively, but I couldn't see at the time that if Dr Lynn wasn't staying there why I should stay.

***

Now, I laughed as I thought back, and felt embarrassed at some of the things I had done. Dr Lynn had been very patient with me. The next time I went to see Dr Dhanji she explained to me that Dr Lynn had rung her up. "I understand what he means. There is no replacement for him, and many people would not have supported you as much as he has. He admits that it is unfortunate your therapy wasn't finished, but there's no one to take his place and he thinks you know everything you need to."

"I understand where he is coming from, but after twenty years of regular support to go from that to nothing, it's harsh. I appreciate everything he has done, but in one way I wish he hadn't. I feel lost. What happens if I have a crisis? Surely it's better I know someone than no one."

"He has left the name of another consultant in case of a crisis, and he is going to have a word with him." She continued to give me the name, and I sighed. I knew the consultant, as I used to say "Hi" to him in the corridor for years when he regularly walked past as I was waiting to see Dr Lynn, and I had known his lovely wife, a nurse at the hospital who had sadly passed away since. She had made an impression on me, as she had tried desperately to get me to join in on the section of the hospital that did activities for the patients, but I had been too shy. She had been lovely and I was sad to find out that she had been so ill, but had been inspired by her strength and professionalism. I was still in a state of shock about Dr Lynn leaving, and couldn't think straight because of the strength of my emotions. "I won't want to see anyone else, as it would be a backward step, but it's helpful to know I have a contact if needed." I said it quietly.

Dr Dhanji nodded in agreement. "I think you will be fine. You're a pragmatic person," she replied. I smiled at her confidence in me.

I referred to Dr Dhanji as my jet-setting GP, as I had never known anyone travel quite so much. I joked that she had shares in the airlines. I admired her energy and laughed at remembering when she had done a huge bungee jump above the rainforests. She also had a wide-ranging vocabulary and I would sometimes either ask her to explain or look the word up afterwards. I left her surgery often thinking I needed to get out more and live. Her new venture was learning to fly and because she seemed to have travelled and explored the whole globe I joked to her, "Not having shares in the airlines is good enough for you, now you need your own plane." She leaned back in her chair laughing, which made me laugh. Sometimes it would help, as it would lift me when I was feeling stressed and anxious. My diabetes was monitored quite well by Maggie, and I tried to manage it but again my blood counts were all over the place. I either took too much insulin or not enough, and I was finding it difficult to reach the happy medium. Dr Dhanji helped me with managing Menieres disease, which would come and go. My ME lurked in the background, which Dr Lynn had said he thought it was more down to my mental health problems. It was frustrating, but I was learning to manage it. I would also need to ask Dr Dhanji advice for the kids, and sometimes they would come in with me to get their ailments sorted. Dr Dhanji was patient and understanding, and several times I had suffered panic attacks in her room after having to wait in a crowded waiting room. I always thought I had held it together, telling myself not to be so stupid, walked cool, calm and collected into her room, sat down and then literally fallen to pieces. I would suddenly be uncontrollably shaking, unable to speak, gasping for air and fighting to take control of myself. It would be embarrassing. "It's your fault," I said, looking at her. "I was alright until I saw you." We both burst out laughing, but I was still shaking. "New curtains, you have new curtains." I had noticed they were blue. I was so trying to concentrate on anything so I could ground myself. "Yes, you're right." She smiled at me. "Are you OK now?"

I nodded. "Your fault."

She laughed.

I was lucky I had been fortunate to have seen some great doctors. My last doctor before Dr Dhanji had actually written to me to congratulate me on my book. Her name was Dr Louise Ojeicha and although it was only for a short period of time, she had given me encouragement and confidence about my first book. I had intended to write under a pseudonym and had asked her opinion. "No, you don't want to do that. It will help people a lot more if they can relate to you. But it is your decision." I had hesitated and looked at her hard, thinking. All the time I had been certain my identity would not be revealed, but now I suddenly realised she was right. I was passionate about introducing more awareness about mental health issues and I didn't want to feel ashamed about what I had been through. I felt proud that I had come as far as I had, and it would have been hypocritical to hide away under a false identity. At that moment I decided to be open about who I was, and Dr Ojeicha even suggested I stick a small photo of myself in the front of my book. I did, but it wasn't easy, and I would have much rather stuck one of my dog on the page. However, although I was not to know at the time, the many messages I received after my book was published showed she was right. When the book was published I sent Dr Ojeicha, who had left the practice, a copy, and I felt very humbled and privileged to receive a letter from her with such a kind endorsement. I was so proud of it I used it when I published the e-book.

It would probably seem no big deal to many people whether their doctor was nice or not, but in my world every relationship or encounter with people carried so much weight. If someone was slightly rude or ignored me it would have a significant effect. I think I lacked so much confidence that I relied on Dr Lynn and his support much more than I should have done. I think he knew this, and I was partly conscious of it, yet at the same time I had nowhere to turn to build myself up. I was still learning to place trust in myself. As the next few weeks passed, I knew I had to face up to this new challenge and I was determined not to let Dr Lynn or myself down.

CHAPTER TWENTY-THREE – DIGGING DEEP

Dr Lynn had written as usual one of his fortnightly letters to Dr Dhanji and I was reading the copy: 'Obviously in great distress at the news that I am leaving'. I nearly snorted to myself indignantly as I read the line. How dare he? The arrogance of the man! I tackled him at our next appointment.

"What makes you think I would be in great distress just because you are leaving?" I said it more as a statement rather than a question. I was feeling angry and upset.

"Well, you are, aren't you?" Dr Lynn looked at me raising his eyebrows.

"No, not at all," I said stubbornly, frowning at him. He sat back, quietly raising his eyebrows again.

I sank back in my chair. "Yes," I conceded quietly. I held back the tears and sat up defiantly. He laughed and so did I. We both knew I was being difficult and both knew I couldn't help it.

"You'll be okay, Bridge, won't you?" he looked questioningly at me. He said it with such a caring attitude that I nearly crumbled, but I held it together.

"Of course," I wanted to say, but I didn't. "I don't know. I hope so. I'll try my best." My voice was faltering. "I won't see Gary even if I am bad. It would be a backward step." Again I fell silent and we both sat there a while. "If I am not my best, it won't be my fault. I will try my hardest and I never quit." I said it with such force. I was trying to convince myself more than him. He nodded and went silent. I noticed he was biting his nails, and in all the years I had known him I had never seen him do it with such force. We sat quietly and I felt sad. "It's alright for you," I said. "Because you knew you were leaving. You planned this, it is a shock to me."

He looked at me and leaning forward he said. "No, you are wrong, Bridge. I didn't know that long ago, and it was a surprise to me." Our eyes met and I stared hard at him. I knew he was telling me the truth. I didn't want to know the circumstances, whether the surprise was an opportunity he took or whether he was forced. I held him in such high esteem and the ending of our professional relationship was very painful, as it had come so unexpectedly either way I wouldn't have been happy. Yet in another way I also wanted him to be happy whatever the decision. I left the appointment struggling again to come to terms with our departure.

February turned into March, and I received a surprise message from Denny, my younger sister. She asked if I would go with her to take Mum to Belgium. I rang her up. "What dates are you looking at? It's so strange, as I had been thinking of asking you the same thing." I laughed and so did Denny.

"I was thinking of mid-May, not June, as I have my charity cycle ride to Skegness," she replied.

I looked at the calendar. "What about 17th May? It's a Friday and we could come back the Monday. I would need to check with Joseph but I think it's a possibility."

"Sounds good. Will you check the fares and ways as I want to drive there. I thought of going through Calais?" Denny replied.

"Leave it with me. I will message you." I put the phone down and Googled travelling from the UK to Belgium. It seemed the Eurotunnel was the most convenient way for Mum, as she couldn't walk far. I did hesitate, as when the tunnel was first built I had always said there was no way I was going under the sea. I wanted Mum to see my aunt, as they had always been close, and Aunty Anita was now in her late eighties. Whereas she and my cousin Vicky had always come to visit us in the past, the last couple of years they hadn't managed it, and it seemed fair for us to make the effort to visit them. Mum had osteoporosis and a hip replacement, and was in pain quite a lot. She had been to the pain management clinic and had been on morphine, yet it still hadn't helped. Although she was on another medication she still suffered, so to take her away for a few days was significant. Denny and I conversed, resulting in us booking the Eurotunnel for the 17th May. It was only a week or so later after I finished with Dr Lynn, so I thought it would be a positive move, acting as a diversion, as I hardly left the house, and I was happy for both my mum and aunt to see each other. I also looked forward to seeing my relatives, as I was quite close to them all and always managed to have a laugh with them. My dad would have been very happy, as it was his brother who had married a Belgian lady, who was my aunt.

I was very close to Aunty Anita. She was a Capricorn like me, and loved animals. She still rode her horse right up to her mid-eighties, and still boarded dogs for other people. She was also my godmother, and I felt fortunate, as we had got on so well. Her sister Colot had made a big impression on me when I was little, as she had four big German Shepherd dogs that used to race to the big iron gates and bark at us as we entered to make our annual visit. She used to shout, "They are fine. Come through!" When you have four massive guard dogs barking at you standing higher than you when they were on two legs, it was a little intimidating, but once inside the garden they were very soft and good-tempered. Denny and I used to skip down her long garden to see the sheep at the bottom and the odd chicken running around. We were too young at the time to realise that the sheep were for the freezer. One of our favourite visits was to visit the Lion of Waterloo. Denny and I would race, climbing all two hundred and twenty six steps to get to the top first. The lion was made of the battle-shells from the Battle of Waterloo, 18th June 1815. We stood in awe, thinking of the bloodshed and glad we were not there at the time. Once at the top we had a fantastic view of Brussels and the surrounding area. My dad was very proud of his Belgiam connections, and worked hard to keep the family together. When I had written *A Fine Line,* my aunt and cousins bought copies and I had been glad I could share my past with them. They never came back to me or questioned me about anything, and once again I felt dejected and also rejected. It took me a long time to come to terms with the fact that no one in my family really was interested in what had happened to me. Only now, four years later, are pieces of my jigsaw starting to slip into place.

CHAPTER TWENTY-FOUR,
REJECTION AND ACCEPTION

When I was younger I was hungry for acceptance. Whether it was from being adopted or genetic make-up, I am not sure. I personally believe it was a combination of social circumstances and my own genetics that formed my personality, behaviour and characteristics. I was and still am sensitive, so the slightest sign of rejection could manifest into a stronger perception than it really was. Looking back, as with a child learning through repetition the difference between right and wrong, I learned that the slightest rejection lead to dejection and non-acceptance. I lacked confidence from when I was very little and being a middle child may not have helped the cause. My mum and dad were so thrilled at being able to adopt after having been told they could not have children that my oldest sister would have been like a forbidden treasure when she was adopted and brought home. As like a diet once you have been denied something for so long when you get chance to have it, you relish in the pickings. Then I came along and apparently even as a baby in the pram would be content, not making a noise, and my mum would say people didn't believe I was there. I was so well behaved that I needed little attention and effort. I think just as I reached the age of awareness and actually needed the attention, my parents were delighted to find out that my mum was pregnant, and this was like having unexpected access to the pot of gold at the end of the rainbow. When Denny was born the attention turned to her, and my shyness increased and I became introverted. I had a great love of animals, and I grew up turning my attention to nature and wildlife more than people. Whilst most of my friends' walls were covered with posters of pop stars, mine were covered with animal portraits with the odd one of a pop star. As I was so shy I didn't demand attention, and consequently sank more and more into the background. By the time I was twelve I was easy pickings for any paedophile and sadly that became the case.

At the time I didn't realise I was being groomed, and although the grooming held such detrimental consequences, in another way it also gave me some confidence. For the first time ever I was led to believe I was important and that what I wanted in life was important. Although I loved my parents and I am sure they only wanted the best for me, they often ignored my wishes and went with their own opinions. I went through a period of intense grooming from Sandra. I believed my parents were wrong to favour my younger sister, and I believed they were against me. I turned to my predator, increasingly wanting to believe that I was worth more and that I deserved better. My ever-present hunger for attention was satisfied, and I didn't have to look for it: waves of attention were thrown at me, and as my confidence grew I started to believe in myself. At the same time I believed every word my predator was telling me. Soon Sandra became like a goddess to me. I worshipped the ground she walked on, I craved her attention and with her encouragement I started to see the worst in my mum and dad.

I soon started to make comparisons, and as the attention swamped me I saw every little detail that my mum and dad did not give to me, and also compared to what they did give Denny. My little sister became an extrovert, and was full of confidence. Although I didn't realise it at the time, my emotions were being used and manipulated, and I turned to my predator to receive praise. I also learned to look out for every mistake my parents made. They were under scrutiny, and my predator made sure I didn't miss any fault, and inside I had a ball of hurt and resentment festering and eating away at me. My predator looked after my nan, who I loved very dearly, and also remonstrated when my parents let her down. She was always very pleasant and nice to my parents, and I wanted her to be, as I wanted my mum and dad to love her as much as I had grown to. By the time I was thirteen years old, my predator and her family had accepted me as one of theirs. Her mum and dad spoilt me, in ignorance of the true situation.

My predator – or Sandra, as I should call her – also fed on my emotions about my biological mother, and soon I was so screwed up internally from the intense grooming and the fact that I had been introverted and vulnerable at the beginning that I needed an outlet for my emotions. Reflecting back, I think that is when I started to self-harm. The fact that Sandra had also started to inappropriately touch and kiss me caused more damage, and without realising it at the time I would sink into dark periods of depression where I just yearned for my biological mum. I suppressed awareness of any inappropriate action, and I was soon in deep denial. I accepted what my mind wanted to accept and I rejected the rest. The additional pressure of exams at a school that had substandard teaching and an appalling record of education and support sent me spiralling down, and the one thing that kept me going was wanting to find my real mum and my love of animals. My parents had let me have my own cocker spaniel at the age of thirteen, and I used to take her on long walks down the park, and used to bird watch and record the different songs of birds on a tape recorder. I lost myself in bird books and dog books, and could soon identify hundreds of the species. I also started to read any books on nature that I could find. I sketched and drew more and more.

Due to the fact that at school no one picked up on the self-harm even though there was clear evidence, especially in physical education lessons where the cuts were clearly visible, and my mum was ill advised to ignore it, I continued to be abused and screwed up. I ended up getting a job in a bank following my parents' wishes, as they did not want me to work in boarding kennels. In their opinion there was no future in it, and they thought the bank was a decent job. I was unfortunate to land in a branch where half the staff were at war with the other half, and being the newest recruit I was picked on depending on which side I made friends with. The attitude of the branch got so bad that transfers were made, and as unsettling as it was, I was transferred to another branch. The manager had come to our branch and picked me out. Little did I know that I was to be once more made a target, and his grooming preyed on my attempt to find my biological mum. His acceptance of me and his attention bought my trust. I thought he was wonderful as he went out of his way to let me use his office to see a counsellor and he supported every move I made. I had moved in with Sandra, still being blind to the true purpose of her attentions. I thought I had made a best friend, and to me she was a cross between a best friend, a sister and a mother. When the bank manager had been nice, it was comforting to know I had support. The day I stopped behind in his office and he raped me was immediately suppressed, and the same day I had been given my biological mum's letter of explanation. Through the different events outlined in *A Fine Line*, I can now look back and see how and why I was unfortunate to fall victim several times to sick predators. I can see why I thought they were helping me, as at the time due to the social circumstances and my deep vulnerability I did not and was not capable of understanding the true abuse. The intense grooming and repetition of grooming kept me in such deep denial and suppression that even when I was being raped it was emotionally blocked off. I concentrated on the social side of the bank. It was a social side that I had not had before, and every member of the staff soon became like family. As the clock was ticking, my perception of true love and friendship was being thwarted. I still loved my mum and dad, but had fallen in love with the wrong people and at the same time my understanding of relationships was being turned upside down. Due to the intensity of the abuse that continued to increase, and unluckily for me the people who I met who took advantage (such as the bank manager and then his wife who succeeded in persuading me to take a lethal overdose that should have killed me), my understanding and vulnerability was like that of a child. I still loved and wanted to see the bank manager's wife even after the medics told me I should have been dead. At the young age of seventeen she had persuaded me to take an additional bottle of paracetamol. I was then unfortunate again, so the severity of the abuse went on continually for well over twenty years and I also survived several murder attempts. There was a serious breakdown of trust through some very sick predators and lack of support from others, because the grooming had not only led me to be isolated but I was also in denial. Even the few close friends and relatives I had were blind to the abuse, which led to me not only self-harming for a release of emotions, as I didn't consciously even realise anything was wrong, but also to also seeing people in a very different light. For many years during the abuse I still worshipped Sandra, and I was unlucky enough to move from job to job involving different predators and sex offenders. By the time I was in my mid-thirties, I was so ill through suppression and denial of the abuse that I had become truly introverted. I had continued to survive as an existence rather than living. The end of the abuse occurred through a car accident and loss of memory which led me to see Dr Lynn.

So strong was the grooming that it was only through medical intervention and a lot of persuasion from Dr Lynn that all connections with Sandra were severed. At this time I was sectioned in hospital and I still could not see that anything was wrong. I denied that the events had happened to me. I could only see that they had happened to 'someone else'. If Dr Lynn questioned or challenged any bad event of my past, I would answer back, "Yes, but you don't understand", and repeat only the good things. This challenging went on for twenty years and even as I write this I have never verbally accepted that there had been anything wrong. This book is another major step into accepting that the people in my past were paedophiles and sex offenders. *A Fine Line* was written in denial, and although I used 'Bridget' – which is actually my middle name – my book *A Fine Line* became a tool to help me stay in denial. It became another angle for Dr Lynn to challenge.

CHAPTER TWENTY-FIVE ACCEPTANCE

Many of the names in *A Fine Line* were changed for obvious reasons, since having taken another step forward to being well I can now reveal that Dr Lynn's real name is Dr Trevor Friedman, and I know that without his professional intervention and support I would not be here now to continue my story.

"Lees, is my name in the new book going to be Dr Lynn, or will it be Dr Friedman?". We both looked at each other and I answered back as truthfully as I could.

"I know it caused me a dilemma, as part of me wanted to write 'Lisa' and reveal many true names. I would have been proud to use your real name from the start, but many of my readers will be used to 'Dr Lynn' and 'Bridget'. If I can use our real names at a later stage, I will." I shrugged my shoulders.

"How far are you in the book now?" Dr Friedman asked.

"Around three-quarters, at a guess. I don't plan anything and write it as it comes. I am still not sure if it has enough material, but I shall write it and see." I hesitated. I was so mixed up with this book. *A Fine Line* had been written on auto-pilot, and although it had been a bestseller, and still is, I was pretty sure it was the uniqueness of the events that had sold it. I had received so many messages from people applauding my courage, and although I felt humbled and thankful, I still felt it was under false pretences. The book was true, but because I was in denial and had written it on auto-pilot I hadn't felt I needed any strength to put the words down. I had written it with no feelings. This book was so much harder, as it was about coming to terms with the past. It was about learning to manage rejection and dejection, denial suppression, and the most important in my mind: acceptance. I think acceptance was the hardest step, as to accept meant coming to terms. Denial was easy; it just kept the pain down. If I accepted what had happened, it opened the door to managing all the other consequences that came with child abuse. It meant I could start to explore my own feelings, and whereas in the past if I perceived someone had rejected me, I would lose confidence, self-esteem and sink into a depressive state, I could now look at it with a new light. Already I felt less of a victim and more of a survivor. I could start to understand why I experienced such feelings. I realised that due to the vulnerability and past experience that I had allowed minor gestures to carry much more weight than was justified. An example would be if my next-door neighbour, who happened to be a friend, rode by my house and looked the other way, it didn't mean she was trying to ignore me or reject me, making me feel dejected. It could have meant she was looking at something that had caught her interest in the opposite direction. If my friend didn't text or ring that week, it didn't mean she had fallen out with me; she could have just been busy. I started to realise that because I had denied all the bad things that had happened and only tried to concentrate on the good parts, it had denied me understanding many irrational feelings that were natural because of the irrational treatment I had received. It had been understandable, because I had been treated so badly that I thought everyone else would do the same. As I couldn't see it, I couldn't also see the irrationality of my own behaviour.

I also started to realise that assuming no one is trustworthy and thinking all are bad had pulled the curtains across and blacked the light out of my social world. I had automatically questioned and anticipated people's moves and motives. Always suspecting the dark side first, this in turn led to a dark world. Now, even as I questioned whether it was necessary to make such judgements, already the curtains had opened just that tiny gap, and a flicker of light was seeping through. Maybe if I could build on this trust I might be able to find a whole roomful of sunshine.

I was a little concerned, as I had just realised that I had started to accept the past, and that I had suffered terrible abuse for over twenty years. I had felt emotions about the murder attempts, spiralling into deep depression, and felt suicidal that people actually wanted me dead. The bank manager's wife had caused me to feel physically sick. I couldn't get my head around the fact that she knew her husband was raping a seventeen-year-old and had done nothing about it except to encourage it to satisfy her own needs and then encourage that same girl to end it all, telling her she hadn't taken enough pills and that she had to take more. Those actions are impenetrable to me, yet I was comforted by how other people reacted when they heard the truth. They were also feeling sick, and it helped me understand that the bank manager's wife's action was extreme and inhuman.

I wished I was still seeing Dr Friedman, as I had so many more questions to ask. He had told me I knew it all. I realised a first in my psychology degree was possibly helping me to manage the acceptance, as I was analysing everything through a clinical aspect. I was questioning responses and behaviour, and had analytical emotions. Although I had accepted the past, I wondered if I had accepted the whole past, as I I still felt nothing at all when I remembered some of the abuse and the physical rapes. It was still blocked, and whether it will still surface, only time will tell. Accepting the past was not easy, because before I could tell myself that in not verbally agreeing to it, the past could still be unreal and like a dream. I could explain all my reasons not to accept it. The main reason was because I was too scared to. When I was in hospital, I had acted out in many ways, and if someone told me beforehand I would carry out such actions, I would have put my life on it that I would never do such a thing. Each time I had acted out I had felt such intense despair that the only way to escape was through irrational actions that were extreme but were impulsive and unplanned.

***

Flashback:
She was being nice to me, and she laughed. "Come on, you. Let's go and get a drink." I followed her into the ward kitchen and we used the boiling water from the gigantic urn to make two coffees and returned to my room. "I wish you were on this ward permanently," I said.
She smiled and replied, "No you don't. You'd get sick of me."
I smiled back and shook my head. Alec was in her thirties and was one of the nicest nurses I had met. She always smiled and was cheerful. She was caring, and as she patted my shoulder I felt like crying. I wanted to kill myself at that moment because the pain was so intense; her being so kind and nice hurt like mad. I looked at her. She had short brown hair and bright blue eyes, and her cheeks bore dimples when she smiled. You could not help but smile back. She was slender and fit; we had gone on a run together and my intentions of showing a high level of fitness were squashed as I panted trying hard to keep up with her. Most of the nurses had a job to keep up with me, but Alec could outrun me any day.
She was also very good at her job, and I could not try anything even if I wanted to. She gave me no chance, and in return I felt safe and respected her. The time changed to the hour, and reluctantly Alec got up to go. "I am here tomorrow. Don't you do anything stupid." I shook my head and smiled as she left the room and the next nurse came to sit with me. I was left feeling extremely low. I wanted to run and cut; I wanted to smash. I wanted to scream my head off. When she had smiled and cared about me, it had hurt more than any words could describe. I was in a mood and I didn't ask my unsuspecting nurse if we could go for a walk. I just got off my bed and walked out of my room. She followed. I walked up to the laundry room where the sheets were stored, and noted there was a ladies' belt off a dress on the radiator. I had used to look for all the rubber seals that went around the bins, but since I had tried to strangle myself a few times with

them, they had been removed. I noted where the dress belt was and walked towards the kitchen. I wanted to see which other nurses were around and where. I made myself and my level-one nurse a drink, and went back to my room. I sat feeling agitated and sipped my tea, trying to ground myself. "When we have finished our drinks, can we go and get a clean towel?" I asked. She nodded, and as soon as I had finished my drink I was up walking towards the laundry room. I passed the radiator with the belt without reaching for it, but on the way back I paused by the radiator and, laughing, said to the nurse, "Looks like you've made the beds again." She laughed and looked across to the dormitory where I pointed, and within a couple of seconds I had taken the belt and hidden it under my towel. We walked back to my room and I felt a glow of satisfaction: not only had I completed a challenge, I was now prepared to strangle myself.

***

Looking back, it is sick that I was so excited and happy about the prospect of being able to strangle. I knew that I hadn't wanted to die. I knew that I hadn't thought things through, and at no time had I thought this could kill me or cause permanent damage. I had two young children that I loved dearly, but at no time had I thought of the more serious consequences. I could remember back and nearly experience the feelings that I had felt at the time. I had felt such an intensity of despair that I needed an extreme reaction to remove it. First the challenge had helped, as it brought and introduced adrenalin and I got fired up. The anticipation of strangling myself caused stimulation, excitement and anticipation. I wondered whether if I had been told, "OK, just go ahead", whether all this would have been removed.

***

Flashback:
Time for bed, and I already had my belt half under my pillow. My level-one nurse sat at the door, nose in her magazine. I was so excited. I was trying hard to contain myself. Heart beating rapidly, brow perspiring, I fingered my weapon. It was a cotton belt about thirty inches long and an inch wide. I slowly pulled it from the pillow and like a slithering snake proceeded to wrap it around my neck. My sheets camouflaged my actions and soon I was able to start tightening the noose. As it tightened I started to feel the familiar throbbing in my neck, which intensified, and the worst pain became from behind my eyes. They felt they were going to bulge out of my head. By this stage and experience I had already worked the noose so it tightened itself. I was at the stage of no return, and even if I had wanted to shout out or ask for help, I'd gone past the stage of capability. I must

have passed out, and the next thing I knew was that a bright light was shining in my eyes and the room was full of nurses. I felt a nick on my neck and a sharp burn as the offending weapon was pulled quickly out of the way. I started to cough and gasp, trying to catch my breath as a doctor turned me into a recovery position. It had been close, but once again I had survived.

***

Reflecting back, I realised how lucky I had been and how intense the feelings were – a trigger from a nurse being kind. It shocked me as even now I still have those feelings. If someone is kind and nice, I have such a job to deal with it. In another sense it made me feel angry and sad, because someone had interfered with my childhood and had not only robbed me of my childhood but had also taken away precious emotions that should have been joyous experiences, not sad. It made me more determined to try to correct and manage these feelings. Again I wished I could ask Dr Friedman how to manage it. I regretted not being able to work this through years ago, but also believed there was a time for everything. I guessed that if I was still seeing Dr Friedman then the pressure and challenge of not accepting the past might still have been going on. It was as if because there was no challenge I could let a little go. Yet through accepting a little, I still needed many questions to be answered. Dr Friedman may not have had the answers, and I wanted to know why my children could make me so happy yet if someone – a relative stranger or even someone close to me – showed any care, I could go to pieces. I wondered if it was because with my children I could release my feelings but with anyone else I was still so guarded that my feelings became bottled. It again made me think of the Jimmy Savile case and how complex abuse was. Because of the denial and suppression, nothing was straightforward. There were many reasons why it was not discovered sooner – some inexcusable, others explainable. Dr Friedman had not managed to finish my therapy and I felt sad that we hadn't managed to reach the core and the acceptance, yet I knew that because of the dedicated support I was fortunate to have reached the understanding I had. It had given me the strength to take on a psychology degree, to face up to certain facts and to attempt to learn what was going on. One of the hardest issues I had to deal with, which I partly managed but would never be able to understand fully until I had accepted the past, was rejection.

CHAPTER TWENTY-SIX – REJECTION

I, already vulnerable and sensitive to the word rejection ever since I found out I was adopted and one of my school friends at a very tender age had called me a 'bastard'. I had been upset and remember asking my nan what it meant. Her reaction had upset me even more and seemed to reiterate that the meaning was significant. I had always felt rejected by my biological mum, even though it had been explained to me that she had no choice. The local vicar tried to make me feel better by saying that I was chosen, yet knowing that I was chosen because my parents thought that they couldn't have their own children didn't seem to make that statement special. At no time had I ever thought, "My God, they are so lucky they adopted me". Rejection seemed to be feared by many who have suffered abuse. They haven't the self-belief and the confidence to see that they are worth more than how they perceive themselves, so that any insignificant sign that may show an inkling of rejection is self-projected and sometimes exaggerated. One of the consequences of abuse is that the abused believes they could have stopped it and they blame themselves. This knocks down their confidence, and they look for rejection because they expect it. This also ties in with depression, as lack of self-esteem can also lead to depression and potentially minimised social contact. Many of the symptoms all link together, and it is a case of which comes first and how to break the cycle. Reflecting back on the abuse that happened to me, I was fine in the initial years at the bank, as I made many friends and seemed to have a social life. Yet when the bank manager groomed me, whilst I was still being groomed by Sandra, I lost most of my contacts because of the demands made upon me. Years later when some of the bank friends contacted me out of the blue, I was hesitant as I had lost confidence and also scared because of the memories that might surface. Some of the friends had worked with the bank manager and had been shocked by the revelations in the book. I knew that I would need to dig deep to find the courage if I was going to meet up with them. I was not deterred, as I seemed to thrive on challenges.

***

I logged into Facebook to see a new friend request. It was quite a shock to find out it was from a friend from the bank many years ago. I was delighted and accepted the friend request. Claire asked if we could meet up.

"You haven't changed," she told me. "Your book made me laugh so much, especially the bit where you sent Joseph a photo of the goat instead of yourself. I was shocked and can't believe you dared write some of the stuff." I smiled back at her. She was a pretty girl with long red hair that shone in the sunlight.

"I wrote it on auto-pilot so it just poured out. I didn't have to think, so it wasn't hard. Yes, many people found it distressing and shocking, but that's what child abuse is, I suppose."

We both went silent and she continued. "I felt so bad that I hadn't helped you at the time."

"You weren't to know. I didn't even know myself, and if my mum and dad didn't know and my own family and closest of friends, then how could you be expected to know?"

"I didn't really know him, and I am glad I didn't work for him. I felt sorry for Sandra, as she seemed so nice and I am sure she loved you." Claire's words made me feel bad, and at the time confused me. But in all the time I had known Claire I don't think she had ever spoken badly about anyone. We joked and chatted about seeing Dick, who had been assistant manager when I had worked for the bank. I agreed to travel over to Whetstone one night to spring a surprise on him. Dr Lynn was against it, and Maggie was adamant it was a bad idea. I was scared, but then thought I wasn't going to let my past affect my future in a negative way anymore. Claire and I had both made friends with Dick on Facebook, and joked to him with hints to start looking over his shoulder. We did surprise him, and I was full of nerves as we entered the pub. We hadn't seen him for thirty years, yet we spotted him straightaway and nearly ran over to tap him on the shoulder before he could turn around and see us.

"Bloody hell!" He laughed at us. "Bloody hell!" We hugged and kissed, and he beckoned us to sit down whilst he got a round in. We both laughed as we sat at the table, and all we could hear was "Bloody hell". The last time I had seen Dick was at the bank, and he had worn a pale green suit and he'd had a mop of red hair. Now he wore a striped polo top and had lost most of his hair, but he still had the same grin and twinkling eyes, and I was happy that we had made the effort to go over and see him. We had a great night, and I was glad that I hadn't let my fear of flashbacks prevent the event. Dick had read my book and was upset by the whole thing. He threatened to string the bank manager up if he ever saw him again. I knew there was no chance, but it made me feel good that they cared about what had happened to me. In some ways the evening helped me put some ghosts to rest. I didn't have to look at the whole bank as an evil place. I was proud that I hadn't rejected my friends because of the past they were linked to. I returned to see Dick again, and this time we met up with an old boyfriend of mine who had also worked at the bank, and who I had stopped seeing because of demands from Sandra. Although I had been dreading meeting them all from fear of triggers and flashbacks, the positivity helped change my thoughts and also helped put some of the feelings into perspective.

***

I started to gain more confidence from accepting the past and from being able to access more memories and thoughts instead of blocking them off. I found out that I was also able to analyse more material, which in turn gave me a greater understanding. This sounds trite, but it was significant because the amount of understanding had so much depth that it gave me access to a more positive outcome because of the benefits it carried. The cycles that had carried so much negativity such as lack of confidence, low self-esteem, and no social contact, leading to rejection, dejection and depression, now started to turn the other way. I could understand that the rejection lay more in my mind than with the other person, I gained confidence, my self-esteem grew and my social contacts increased. My depression started to lift and slowly but clearly I could see more light filtering through to my life.

CHAPTER TWENTY-SEVEN –
STANDING ON MY OWN TWO FEET

It was turning into April and I felt despondent when I went to see Maggie, my diabetic nurse. "What's up?" she asked, and I couldn't even answer. It was dawning on me that I might never see Dr Friedman again, and he had been like a best friend. I did confide a lot to my friends, yet I didn't see them that much. I struggled with the pressure at home, and Dr Friedman had been my support and outlet. It was rare for Joseph to ask me how I had got on. I don't think he was being mean; it was just that he took it for granted that I was OK, and to be honest even if I wasn't I would rarely tell him. Dr Friedman was so professional he could challenge my thoughts where most people couldn't reach. He was still challenging me about the past, and now that we had a time limit he was pushing harder. However, I just closed down even more. It was ridiculous, because he and I knew that my reasoning was so perverse at times. He told me and I knew, but I still couldn't stop myself. Now as I faced Maggie I couldn't speak.

"Look, you have to pull yourself together. You have two children. He isn't worth it." She was telling me off at the same time as looking at my blood counts. "These are high, aren't they? I suppose in the circumstances it's not surprising." I nodded, as I knew that I hadn't been monitoring my sugar counts as well as I could have done. "You will be OK, I know you will." She smiled at me and I knew that she was right, but I felt like I was grieving and I just couldn't cheer up. The following week I developed a sore throat and a cough, but as usual I ignored it hoping I wasn't catching the virus that Jo Jo had suffered from the previous week. Suddenly I seemed to go downhill so quickly it took me by surprise, and within a day I was bedridden. My temperature went up to 40 and my diabetes was so high I had to increase my insulin by ten times more. I knew Dr Dhanji was away, so I checked with Maggie by phoning her. I had great difficulty in talking and I squeaked and croaked rather than spoke, then my voice would go so high. Maggie told me I had to check and inject every two hours, and soon I felt like a pincushion, but I accepted the importance of keeping my sugar levels steady. I monitored every hour, as the massive increase in insulin was so unbelievable I was worried about having hypos. My temperature did not go down, and my voice was nearly nonexistent. I rang Dr Dhanji the first chance I got, and she had difficulty in understanding me with my voice so bad. She prescribed antibiotics, and told me I had severe laryngitis and flu. It was to be another week before I could stand up and another few to recover. I was hoping that I would be alright to travel to Belgium, and my other thoughts were that I didn't want to miss seeing Dr Friedman as I had only ever missed one appointment in the twenty years and that was because of a funeral. Being ill was unpleasant, but it was also a lesson to appreciate what I had when I was well.

It was the last but one appointment with Dr Friedman, and we both seemed on edge and laughed about one more to go. It had been a sad few months, because not only was Dr Friedman retiring from the NHS but the hospital wards had been transferred to another area in Leicester. Slowly but surely I had seen many people who had become close acquaintances through seeing them every other week over the last twenty years disappear to the other hospital. I felt quite privileged that so many came up to give me a hug as I waited in the corridor for Dr Friedman to come down. The receptionist gave me a massive hug and told me to take care, and cleaners came over, along with many of the nurses. The last few weeks had been hard, as each time I had visited the hospital there were fewer and fewer people there. The gloomy building became even darker as the superficial lights were turned off one by one. The doors that had once been active and swinging open were locked, and footsteps echoed even louder in the empty corridors. Although sad, it seemed fitting that the hospital unit was to close, because Dr Friedman and I were also leaving to make new journeys elsewhere. Today we sat facing each other and surprisingly enough I was quite calm. The last few weeks I had insulted him so much. Again he had asked if I would be OK, and I had answered, "What do you care? It won't make any difference. In a few weeks as you won't be paid to ask." The last time I had added, "Next you'll be giving me the last final dates." It had been a coincidence, but he held out a slip of paper with the last three dates on and had also told me to "Fuck off". I had deserved it, as deep down I knew he cared and that he had given me the dates so I could come to terms and accept them better. We reminisced and laughed about some of the incidents that had happened in the hospital. I also told him about an incident with my mum.

"She turned around to me and said, "Do you miss the bank?". It came from nowhere, and she continued, "I am glad you took after me." My mum had worked in the bank. "It was the best setting and start you could have had."

Dr Friedman looked genuinely shocked. "And how did you reply? Or wasn't it worth it?" His last remark made me realise that he understood that my mum was in her eighties and she didn't realise the hurt inflicted by her words. I had been severely raped, abused and nearly lost my life through the bank. I should have died too, as the overdose was well over the lethal limit. "It wasn't worth it." I smiled at him and felt sad because it had been comforting that he understood the hurt, and I felt I had no others to turn to. I did have virtual friends on Facebook, who meant so much to me and we supported each other, yet the comfort wasn't the same as a face-to-face meeting. If my mum and sisters had just given me a little understanding, my recovery would have been helped along so much. The fact that Dr Friedman had showed he cared so much had given me back some faith in others, and so had Dr Dhanji and Maggie and all the previous medics who had helped. Some of my friends had too, but it was the support from my family that I needed most and it just wasn't there. Again it is sad, but I am not alone. Many sufferers from child abuse do not receive the support from loved ones – it seems to be another tragic consequence of the event. It does hurt and slows down recovery, but sufferers have to accept it is not because loved and close ones do not want to react and respond. The nature of the fate seems to make it so difficult that they genuinely are so close that they are incapable without support for the appropriate response. They take the easiest route and denial comes into force. The most important aspect is to not let that become another negative to weigh one down, and to accept that it is not personal. It is just another factor that is manageable if it is accepted that this seems universal. The same response with my book: I received thousands of messages – some from worldwide – yet the closest people to me remain unresponsive due to the nature and subject of the book. Dr Friedman had also helped me with this and pointed out that many people would not change and although painful, to recover was to accept it and move on. I had come to realise that I had to stand on my own two feet to make a fuller recovery.

"Well, what will you do?" he asked me smiling gently.

"I'd like to try to write, but I am not sure really," I replied. I felt like asking him what he would do in his spare time, but I knew this was out of our remit. He could ask me personal questions as it related to my health and had been necessary in the past. Our relationship was professional, but after twenty years it was nearly impossible not to care about the other person, and I did care about him. I looked at him, thinking about when I first met him and how good-looking and striking he had been then. He still looked good now: instead of his dark hair and moustache, his silvery grey hair gave him a distinguished look and his tall lean figure carried an air of charisma with a hint of arrogance. I respected him, yet we had been through a great deal and I wasn't afraid to speak my mind.

The appointment flew by, which seemed strange, as already I was holding back. I realised I had done so since I had found out he was leaving. In one way there seemed not much point in telling him my worries about the children or personal problems, as although he had helped in the past, it wasn't going to be a great deal of help now. Invisible boundaries had already started to appear, and it was as if I was putting an internal guard up and reverting back to my old self. I used to believe that keeping everything to myself was being tough, as then only I could hurt myself, no one else. I had now learned that this was a lonely route and to be better I had to make the effort of socialising more and trusting others. It wouldn't be easy, but I knew I owed it to myself to give it a go. I followed Dr Friedman out through the dark waiting room, having a quick glimpse at the notice board where I could still see information about my book on display. He held the door for me and then he went upstairs as I took the downstairs route. "Thank you," I said, as I always did, before running down the stairs into the light.

Since Dr Friedman had informed me he was leaving, my thoughts had been thrown into disarray. I was used to routine, and after twenty years my thinking process had suddenly changed. I had always planned and aimed towards the next appointment. It wasn't in the forefront, but I knew I had a date where if I was struggling I could attempt to hold off any negativity until I saw him. Now I wasn't settled: part of me was trying to ignore or avoid any upset, and the other half of me was telling myself not to worry and that I could deal with it. I felt like I was a storage disk being defragmented, so that all my little pieces of thoughts were being organised and arranged in order to eventually function better, but at the present time it was a bit confusing. Another part of me was thinking positively that I was better I didn't need to have therapy. Another part was telling myself what a load of...

This hadn't been planned. It was down to circumstantial events that my therapy had been cut short. I could choose a negative pathway and start to complain, shoot my mouth off and decide I was a victim, or I could take the opportunity of using the circumstances in a positive way. I was attempting to do the latter, and I kept thinking of all the people who had sent messages to me in the past when they had been struggling, and hadn't had the good fortune of receiving any support, or if they had it had been little. I so wanted to stand on my own two feet and knew I would try my hardest.

It was strange, because as my last appointment with Dr Friedman drew closer, I started to think of my dad and also of Martin, our neighbour and friend. I travelled into town with Tee Jay and spoke to him. "It's my last session with Dr Friedman next week," I said, concentrating on the road.

Tee Jay replied. "Not good. Why can't he still see you, Mum, out of hospital hours?" I laughed and smiled. "It doesn't work like that, and anyway it had to finish at some stage. It's just because I haven't many male friends who I can rely on. My dad – your grandpa – isn't here, and Martin I don't see that much, and I am just a little sad." I sighed a deep sigh. Here I was already talking to my son as if he was a grown-up, and he was only fourteen years old. "Never mind. It will be a good thing not to have to travel to the hospital." We drove on in silence.

Tee Jay was growing up so quickly and he was so caring. I hoped when he got married he would meet the right girl who would be as kind back, not someone who would take advantage of him. I thought of Martin and why he had meant so much. I hadn't met him or Joyce – or Joanie, as he called Joyce – until I had moved to where we were now. Even then it was a few years before we got to know them, and Joyce had been kind enough to visit me when I was in hospital. She had become a really good friend and had helped me through the dark periods. She was one of the very few people who did want to listen and did care, and where most would be embarrassed or turn their backs she had got involved and had been upset when she had seen me on my darker days. She also had so much sense, and was very practical. Martin her husband had also befriended me and had cared so much that he, like Joyce, had taken the time out to read my book, and he had been supportive. Joyce had even let me stay one night at their house when I was on the run from the police. I had absconded from the hospital, and she had driven by me walking a mile or so from home. I hadn't wanted to be at home, because I was so ill, but I had also needed a break from the hospital and Joyce had driven back to pick me up and they let me stay for the night. Joseph and I had been to London a few times with them, and Martin had taken me to the opera once when Joyce was busy. We had some fun times. I cared about both of them a lot.

I did feel depressed, as I was thinking my dad had gone, I hardly saw Martin now and Dr Friedman would be retiring. It was a bit out of perspective, as I loved my dad but we were on different wavelengths when it came down to my personal problems. I just missed him. I loved Joseph but we didn't talk enough, and when we did we didn't always agree. I talked to Tee Jay a lot, but again I was very aware of his age and there was a balance of being truthful but of also being protective.

One of the people who had also helped me a lot was Paula. I had met Paula when she was a Homestart volunteer. We had been introduced when I had just moved to the area, and she had become a very good friend of the family. It had taken me years to trust her, and in turn she had been very patient with me. I had questioned her motives and her reasons. I used to write to her every week. I had used this method with Dr Friedman and remember posting letter after letter. When I used to visit him I would not sit and talk, but sit there quietly and reach hesitantly into my bag to give him sheets of written messages. Paula was now regarded as one of the family and although she had retired from Homestart she still visited us. We as a family valued her friendship a lot. I was also very lucky to have a good friend called Gail who I had met through the school days, and it was on social outings with Gail that taught me how important it was to make the effort to go out and have fun.

It was the big day. I had woken up feeling sick and was dreading going there for the last time, and these feelings already told me how I felt. I did not feel happy in any way that it was my last visit. I called in to see my mum and acted normal, not wanting her to know because I knew I would not handle her reaction very well. I also did not let onto the kids and Joseph. I wanted minimal fuss.

As I waited in the corridor, Dr Friedman walked through on time. We both smiled at each other as we walked through the door into the room. "Well, this is it, Lees," he said as he sat down. I nodded and arranged my coat and bag as I had always done, and sat down facing him. There seemed little point in bringing up the past, as our sessions were ending. "How's the book going?" he asked.

"Well, we need to hurry up and finish this session, then I can finish my book," I replied. We both laughed. It seemed a strange coincidence that I was finishing my account of my past and that Dr Friedman and I were finishing our sessions. Life worked in mysterious ways sometimes.

"I am a little worried about going to Belgium, as the last time I went with Denny was thirty-two years ago and I ended up in hospital for going down the stairs. I hope it doesn't give me any serious triggers as I won't have any back-up," I stated.

"Why on earth are you going?" he asked, looking at me.

"It was something that had been on my mind. I love my relatives over there, and Mum hasn't been able to travel to see my aunt. When my sister suggested it I thought it would be a good diversion as it is not going to be easy for the first few months after finishing our sessions. I was trying to be positive and hadn't really thought it through. I will not let my mum down now. It will also be a challenge and a test to see how I cope," I smiled at him.

"You have always coped well in pressure, and I have to admire how you have handled this. Many people would come in here feeling anger, being bitter and taking it as an excuse to fall apart. You have come in here smiling, relaxed, and looking how to be positive and cope…"

I interrupted. "Well, there's no point in handling it any other way. It's happening and I have to deal with it." My voice shook and I went quiet. Although I was trying my hardest to stay calm, inside I felt sick.

I had written to Dr Friedman after our previous session saying that I knew with regard to lifestyles he probably lived on another planet to me – I suggested I lived on Pluto, as I had to get my dog theme in, and I reckoned he lived on Venus, and then thought of the famous book and reckoned I had his planet wrong, but was not going to talk to him about that. Yet I had suggested it would be an idea for us to meet up in the future, as I so wanted to show him I could cope without his support. This to me would help in a few ways. It would show he did care about me, although I thought he did. It would motivate me to cope when I was feeling vulnerable and because after all this time I did care about him, I had so much to thank him for. At the same time I still wanted to respect the professional relationship, yet accepted that it was an exceptional situation and sort of saw him as a friend as well. I anticipated that he would tell me off and tell me it was out of the question. I was still a believer in 'if you don't ask you will never know'.

"About my book: I just wanted to say thank you for offer of writing a foreword. I would like you to, but you need to read it first as you might not want to after you have read it. I think the book might not be clinical enough for you." I sighed.

"It is the little personal things readers like to know, like what the night staff get up to," he replied.

"Well, I can only write it and see. I remember when I wrote my first book you asked who would read it, and I said it might only be you but I needed to do it. I never dreamed it would have the response it did." I shrugged my shoulders.

"I think the fact that you did have a response and it showed you that people do care has been helpful."

"Yes, but I also got some nasty reviews that hurt," I said.

"You are always going to have somebody who will oppose. Get used to it, Lees, as these things happen and they are life." He smiled as he said it and I accepted that I still had a long way to go to toughen up.

The session was coming to an end, and I already knew what he was going to say as he looked at his watch. "We'll have to end it there." I looked up to his face and his eyes glistened with tears. I felt very emotional. "This is where we walk out," he said.

I nodded and stood up, but before I reached for my bag I said quickly, " I asked you about meeting up. I know you will say it's a silly idea and…"

"No, Lees, it's a good idea. I would like to see you and know how you are doing. This is an exceptional case and we have known each other for a long time. But it can't be for at least six months or even longer."

"Oh no, I agree. I need to heal and move on first." I smiled. I felt relief, and my sadness lifted. There was a massive difference between saying a final goodbye and knowing I would see him at some stage in the future. It also made me feel good. We hugged and my tears welled up, but I fought them back down. I followed him through the waiting room, along the corridor and to the doors where he would go upstairs and I would go down. "Wait." I impulsively pulled on his arm and he turned round. I put my arms around him and hugged him as tightly as I could. "I love you. Professionally, of course. Thank you," I whispered, and as he smiled and went up the stairs, I turned and headed down the stairs, past the window I had once tried to leap out of, and out of the building into a new era.

EPILOGUE

I did go to Belgium and I was determined to face my fears and to enjoy myself. Denny drove and I navigated, while Mum sat in the back, and we went by the Eurotunnel, a route I had always said I would never take through fear of travelling under the sea. We visited loved relatives who we had not seen for a long time. On the Saturday we went with our cousin Vicky to the Grand Place in Brussels, and travelled by bus. They both laughed at me. "Another first in a long time," Denny said.

I laughed. I hadn't been on a bus for thirty years or more. We then went on the tube, another rare experience, and I still jumped at how fast the doors opened and shut. Arriving in Brussels I was taken back by the flamboyant dressing of the people, who seemed to have a completely different dress sense and culture. Vicky asked, "Is it like this in London?" Denny and I both looked at each other and shrugged our shoulders, mesmerised by the sheer number of people laughing and having fun. We walked around the corner and suddenly Vicky started laughing. Denny and I joined in as we came across a carnival lorry with a massive poster stating 'Gay Parade Brussels 2013'. Vicky, who was slightly older than me but very young for her age, swung back her long hair, her eyes twinkling, and she said, "Well, cousins!" We could not help but enjoy the atmosphere. I looked around, deciding I had been living under a stone for too many years. I couldn't tell who was a she or he at times, but admired the openness, and it was nice to see so many people having fun and enjoying themselves. On the Saturday night Denny and I ended up at a fantastic rock concert with Vicky. Her boyfriend Fil was a member of one of the bands. Denny and I became known as 'the cousins'. We danced into the early hours of the morning and then visited a local market where we laughed like kids sampling a big bag of warm Belgian waffles. "No. Smell first." Denny tapped my fingers and held the bag towards me: they smelt gorgeous and I eagerly bit into one. It was still hot, and it just melted in my mouth. I could have finished the whole bag.

"Glad Maggie can't see me!" I laughed. "Sod the diabetes. I'll behave again later." I limited myself to two, and left Denny and Vicky to finish them. Later we visited my aunt and met my other cousin, and then we said our farewells as we were due back the next day. The trip had been a huge positive for me. It had been unexpected, and Denny and I laughed most of the journey and Mum enjoyed herself. It was a couple of days later when Mum told me it was the best weekend of her life. I decided that I had to start living again and make the effort to do more.

June arrived, and I received an unexpected friend request on Facebook. I was taken aback yet delighted at the same time. It was from my younger biological sister Debbie who I had never had contact from before. I accepted and we started to message each other. Another shock came when we exchanged photographs of our sons, as her son Kurtis was the same age as Tee Jay and they had such a striking resemblance that it was uncanny. Further conversations through messaging revealed they also had very similar characteristics and personalities, including similar skin conditions. It was obviously down to the genetics. I immediately wanted to tell Dr Friedman that my biological sister had been in contact and realised I couldn't. Vicky also messaged me telling me that there had been another rock concert and people were asking where 'the cousins' were. She told me we had received compliments all night and even when one of the bands went on stage they opened their performance with a comment about 'the cousins'. "You were a huge success," she wrote, and it made me smile and reflect that life was precious. Vicky had also chatted to me about my book, and again I realised that I had previously presumed the worst, that my relatives didn't care, but in another perspective, maybe it was having the right opportunity to communicate. I realised I had to think more positively than I had done in the past. Denny texted me yesterday and told me that she would like me to go to Mum's on Friday 14th June for her 50th birthday for tea and cakes in the morning. She also wrote that Jane would be there and asked if it would be a problem. Jane had not spoken to me since I had my first book published, and had cut off all contact with the children as well. I replied back that I would be there. I was nervous about seeing my older sister, but again I knew deep down I loved her very much.

I saw Dr Dhanji this week and she prescribed some medication for my tennis elbow, and as she prepared the prescription, I joked that she hadn't done anything out of the ordinary for a while. I also told her that I was trying to be positive but was still struggling a little. "You need to cheer me up," I said to her, smiling.

"I am having my first flying lesson on Saturday," she replied with a wink.

"Actually, I can't see you in a Cessna, more like a Tornado." She laughed again and as I got up to go she turned around and said, "You will be fine, you know."

I turned on my way out. "Thanks," I said, smiling and shutting the door behind me. I waved to Julie the receptionist and made my way outside. I called in at the chemist to get my prescription and both ladies went to get it together, apologising to each other. "Great service," I joked to them., It was silly things like the little gesture of both ladies trying to help me at once that made me feel good. Dr Dhanji inspired me, as she was so active and always smiling. Maggie made me laugh, yet she was so empathic, friendly and wanting to help. Julie always took time out to greet me. I rushed home to check on my animals and to see if Cadbury the white goat was getting better. He had been so ill and we had nursed him day and night to try to save him. The vet hadn't given him much chance, but they had been brilliant rushing to help as soon as we had called. Cadbury did look a lot better, and I was relieved, as Tee Jay loved him. The kittens ran up to greet me and I laughed as both Cara and Asti shared a bone. Tee Jay would be back soon from school, Joseph was in his office, and Jo Jo was at home revising for her exams. I realised another Tuesday had gone by, and I had managed without seeing Dr Friedman. A friend on Facebook had just messaged asking if I had finished my next book, as she needed a new book to read. I smiled. It was great motivation for me. People had sent messages of thanks and encouragement after my last book, and many said they had been inspired. What they didn't realise was that their own positivity and thanks had helped inspire me a lot too. Many people who had suffered from similar experiences had inspired me so much. Their belief in me helped me cope through the difficult times. Paula had heard snippets from this book, and her feedback was that I had moved on so much and that the insight was amazing. When I told her Dr Friedman had agreed to see me in the future, her words had been, "Well, he proved you wrong. He hasn't let you down and he does care." I smiled. I realised that as long as you believe in yourself and know that people do care, then you have to move forward. One of the biggest skills I had learned was looking on the bright side, of trusting and of letting people in, of opening the door just a little bit to allow a whole new life to begin.

Some of the messages received from readers of *A Fine Line – A Balance to Survive.*

A solicitor who works on a panel for children's welfare:
Lisa - I am going to buy the book so I can read it all! It was painful because it touches so much on what I do. So many people would not even believe the experiences outlined in the book. The descriptions of self-harming are painful to read. So many of my clients go through it. Your book for the first time has made me understand it better. Just by the fact you wrote the book shows that some people can break free and come out of the other end of such experiences. Sadly, many of my clients continue in the downward spiral. Maybe your book will help us professionals to understand how to help them dig themselves out. Well done. We will write a comment in the next few days, but want to think about it.

Dear Lisa. I work as a **psychotherapist/psychologist** with many women who have shared similar experiences to yours. I think they would find hope reading your book...
Thank you for writing...You are inspiring and your work will make a difference to the lives of others... Keep writing...
Thank you for being an inspiration to me and many others! X

June 6th 2012
Hello there, I have read your autobiography. In fact, finished reading it last night, and I must say you are a true inspiration to every being suffering the way you have. I can't even begin to imagine the trauma you experienced on many different occasions but you fought long and hard and not only do you have the love and support from your family and friends, you have 1000s of supporters behind you!! Thank you for sharing your story with us, you are truly amazing! Xxx

Hello, I'm halfway through your book and just wanted to say it's the one and only book I have ever read that seems " real" if you know what I mean. It's messed up, it's not in order, but it makes perfect sense! Thank you for writing it from our point of view. :) You are a brave and lovely lady.

I am reading your book at the moment and think you are a truly inspirational person!!!! I have alot of issues myself that I am trying to work through. I am lucky to have two fabulous nurses who invest alot of time and patience in me. I can only hope I make it through the other side!!! Much love to you and your family xxx

It was quite a moment when I received a copy of this book written by a friend of my daughter. It is the story of her struggle for mental stability after severe trauma and betrayals. She has had to self-publish, despite recommendations from psychiatrists, because 'sob-lit' is said to have had its day. But, 'sob-lit' this isn't. It is, I think, a very important book.

The time when her trauma's were occurring was the 70's. We have come a long way. It was an era when we were extremely careful how and what we spoke to others, especially our elders and those in authority. Reputations were all and the next generation knew what was at stake for older people. The book is a timely reminder that even now some people may not be able to find their voice, in a desperate situation.

The book is very readable: I couldn't put it down I hope it will be well borrowed from our own library, especially by those concerned with training nurses and carers in mental health situations. She quietly gives examples of the comments from both uncaring staff and from those who cared, and thus gave her book her life. The remembered dialogues are so vivid.

I am, however, left with deep sadness and shame that my generation did not notice enough, were not aware.

I think the book belongs in our girardian section in the library as it gives a living example of how humans are afraid to get involved in things-afraid to step outside group-belonging-afraid to upset the applecart: all manifestations that love is embedded in.

By Brenda Wall
Old Middle Foster Home, The Retreat. Yorkshire

About the author Lisa WB

Lisa Whenham-Bossy MBPsS HSC lives in the countryside with her family and animals. She is still passionate about helping other survivors and promoting better understanding into mental health care. Lisa still receives many messages and thanks from her first book A Fine Line and this motivates her to support other survivors where possible.

Lisa will always be grateful for the support and care she received whilst being under the care of Dr Trevor Friedman and still feels privileged to be in contact with him.

Lisa now tries to spend as much time as possible with her children and husband, appreciating the countryside and surrounding area where she has plenty of animals and friends to keep her company.

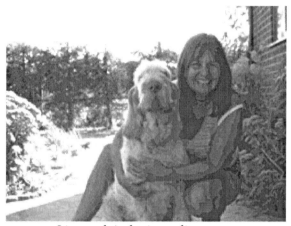

Lisa and Amba in earlier years.

Lightning Source UK Ltd.
Milton Keynes UK
UKOW04f1110310815

257825UK00001B/178/P